Color Healing: A Practical Guide

Graham Travis

Color, in the form of energy waves, accompanies human beings throughout their lives from the moment of conception, through illness and health, in mind and body. Since the body expresses many of its states through changes in skin color, the ancient mystics and healers concluded that color influences people's lives and health, and should be used as a healing factor.

This book discusses the history of the mysticism of color as well as color healing, and explains clearly and simply what healing properties each color contains, and which physical or mental problem can be solved by each color. By using this book, each one of us can take full advantage of the energies of color for our own benefit.

Graham Travis, a physicist by training, is a color therapist who practices in the UK and Europe. Travis' wife, a well-known painter, made him acutely aware of the nuances of color in art. After her tragic death in a traffic accident, he decided to devote his life to color healing and therapy. This book is dedicated to her.

D1465182

ASTROLOG - THE HEALING SERIES

Holistic Healing
Rachel Lewin

Feng Shui
Richard Taylor and Wang Tann

Reiki
Bill Waites and Master Naharo

Bach Flower Remedies
David Lord

Aromatherapy
Marion Wayman

Reflexology
Nathan B. Strauss

Shiatsu
Nathan B. Strauss

Feng Shui for the Modern City
Richard Taylor

Shiatsu for Lovers
Nathan B. Strauss

Color Healing
Graham Travis

Aura-Reiki
Bill Waites

Fifty Massage Points for Self-Healing
Nathan B. Strauss

Color Healing

A Practical Guide

Graham Travis

Astrolog Publishing House

Astrolog Publishing House
P. O. Box 1123, Hod Hasharon 45111, Israel
Tel: 972-9-7412044
Fax: 972-9-7442714
E-Mail: info@astrolog.co.il
Astrolog Web Site: www.astrolog.co.il

© Graham Travis 2000

ISBN 965-494-105-8

Published by Astrolog Publishing House 2000

Printed in Israel
1 3 5 7 9 10 8 6 4 2

CONTENTS

PART 1

What is the Aura?

The aura is the electro-magnetic field that surrounds not only the human body, but also every organism and object in the universe. Most people are familiar with the pictures of the Christian saints, who are portrayed with a circle of golden or white light around their heads; or the angels, who radiate light; or the biblical verse that tells of Moses descending from Mount Sinai with "a ray of light" issuing from his face. These circles and rays are the aura. However, auras do not only surround saints, angels, or ancient leaders. The "holier" a person is - that is, the extent of his energetic purity and his spiritual link to lofty and sublime energy levels - the higher the frequency at which his electro-magnetic field vibrates, creating the sensation of a "radiant" face, or "luminous" eyes. All of us, though, without exception, as well as animals, plants, and objects, are surrounded by an electro-magnetic field to a greater or lesser degree.

For many years, the aura was a concept that was understood mainly by religious figures, thinkers, healers, shamans, clairvoyants, and people with supernatural powers, who could see or feel it. Many ancient sources and books of mysticism discuss the aura and relate to it in various ways.

There is a high consensus among the ancient writings, which reflect various sources and represent most of the peoples of the world in understanding the external and internal influences of the aura, what it symbolizes, as well as its colors and size.

During the twentieth century, with the development of science, increasing numbers of scientists began to take an interest in the mysteries of the electro-magnetic field. Michael Faraday, Nikola Tesla, and Thomas Edison are among the many scientists who came across the electro-magnetic field surrounding the human body in their experiments, and were astounded by their discovery. In the 1940s, many scientists conducted experiments to understand and discover the nature of the electro-magnetic field. The best-known of them was the Russian scientist, S. D. Kirlian (in fact, he and his wife published their research under his name), who developed Kirlian photography, by means of which he succeeded in documenting the delicate energy field that surrounds living organisms.

Today, this method of documentation is called electro-photography. This technique exploits a phenomenon which is called "aura discharge." The aura is the result of the discharge of electrons - millions of electrons are discharged and move toward a special part of a camera, which absorbs them, and according to the structure of the camera and the type of film, astonishingly beautiful color photographs of patterns of energy discharge are created.

In Kirlian photography, hands and feet are generally photographed. The hands and feet are briefly exposed to high-frequency rays that are radiated onto the photographic plate, and the result is documented on photographic paper. After the film is developed, a breathtaking photograph of the electro-magnetic field surrounding the hands or the feet is revealed. Incredibly, the tip of each digit has its own unique electro-magnetic field.

The technique of Kirlian photography evoked many theories involving reflexology and acupuncture. When a particular area of the hand or foot - mainly at the tip of the fingers or toes - had a weak aura, an aura with blockages or holes, and so on - it transpired that the meridian linked to that particular point, or the reflex area (it could be an organ in the body) was also experiencing problems.

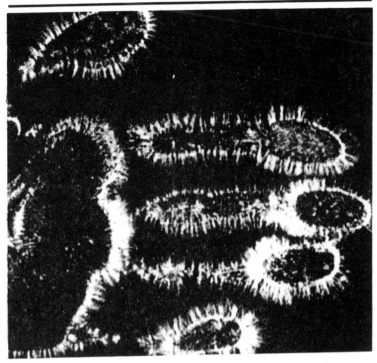

As a result of the development of Kirlian photography, many mysteries concerning our electro-magnetic field gained new and clearer explanations. One of the most astounding things that was understood when this special technique was developed was the "phantom effect." This is a condition in which an amputee feels that he still has his amputated body part. He may feel a kind of itching, prickling, or other sensations in the body part - which in fact is not there! By means of Kirlian photography, it was discovered that when a leaf is cut in two, and each half is photographed using this special method, the electro-magnetic field of the *whole* leaf shows up in the photograph!

This amazing fact was repeated in photographs of amputees, in which it was possible to see the electro-magnetic field outlining the shape of the amputated limb.

When the work of many researchers in the field, especially S. D. Kirlian, was published, interest in the electro-magnetic field and the aura began to grow. Finally, science confirmed what countless mystics, healers, and shamans had known for millennia.

Today, research in the field is gaining momentum, and many researchers are already beginning to examine and apply diagnostic and therapeutic methods using the aura. However, a true breakthrough (and as we will see, it is happening right now) will only occur when the link between the scientific discoveries and cosmic energy is understood more profoundly - an expression, as it were, of the energy that we call "God," "universal force," or any other name with a similar meaning and intention.

Today, the fact that every organism and object in the universe is surrounded by a unique electro-magnetic field is a scientifically proven fact. This electro-magnetic field can be positive or negative, perfect or defective. However, the electro-magnetic field is not something static that is not affected by anything. On the contrary - it is dynamic, variable, and affected by many factors. The organisms in the universe live in a perpetual state of energetic "give and take" between various energetic fields, and they must constantly safeguard their electro-magnetic field from harmful negative or "energy-draining" electro-magnetic fields. Many studies have shown how plants, for instance, curl up when negative or hostile energy (such as pruning shears) is present in the vicinity of their electro-magnetic fields. This is how human beings, too, are liable to feel when in the presence of non-positive energy radiated by places, people, or various objects.

You have no doubt experienced a situation in which for some reason that cannot be explained by your five senses, you have entered a room and felt an uncomfortable and unpleasant sensation, or you have conversed with somebody, and have subsequently felt drained of strength - as if your energy had been "drained" out of you - without being able to explain why. This phenomenon stems from an incompatibility between your auras, or from the fact that one of the auras is too strong and dominant, or from a certain lack of equilibrium that is manifested in the electro-magnetic field. Although most people are not aware of it (many people today, however, have developed or are developing their awareness to the level of understanding and feeling these energetic conditions), this information is absorbed by our electro-magnetic field, which transmits the messages to the nervous system, and affects our general feeling (causing us to feel uncomfortable, rejected, anxious, and so on) - so as to make us get away from the person or place whose energies are incompatible with ours, or are liable to harm us or our energetic equilibrium in some way.

Animals are extremely sensitive to this. While their natural sensitivity is not greater than ours, they operate directly in accordance with their energetic feeling, and react according to the messages they receive. Dogs and cats are able to sense non-positive or incompatible energies wherever they are, or sense, energetically, the quality of the person standing opposite them. The biochemical explanations for those sensations in animals are correct, but constitute merely a part of all the feelings to which animals react (that is, they explain the phenomenon on the biochemical level, which is additional and linked to the energetic level, and not a substitute for it), and only partially explain the phenomenon.

Every person, without exception, is capable of sensing electro-magnetic fields, which are called "auras," and even seeing them to some extent, if he perseveres at developing these abilities. The reason why most people do not see or feel auras is that these senses, like their more physical senses (sense of smell, hearing, etc.) are not sufficiently developed - it can even be said that they are atrophied. However, it must be remembered that this ability can be developed to a greater or lesser extent.

This ability, with its varying levels, does not operate in accordance with simple, familiar physical laws. We are able to pick up energetic messages independently of time and distance. Of course, the ability of the nervous system and the senses to interpret the messages depends on the person's ability to develop his sensitivity to these messages. Telepathic messages, for instance are a pretty clear example of this ability. The principles according to which the various healing and bio-energy methods operate present this ability in a different way.

The structure and function of the aura

As we explained previously, every organism in the universe is surrounded by a unique electro-magnetic field, and there is constant interaction between the electro-magnetic fields of the organisms. Thus, in fact, every person is joined and linked to the environment in which he lives, to the people with whom he chooses to share his life, and to nature - actually, to the entire universe - via this electro-magnetic field.

The question is: How does the aura "function"?

When we relate to this question from the scientific point of view, and according to the activity of the human body, we must remember the well-known fact that an electron that flows, for instance, inside the electrical current of a nerve, causes the flow of electrical energy and of a magnetic field. The electrical current and the field itself are linked to each other, thus creating the electro-magnetic field.

In order to understand and illustrate the *modus operandi* of the magnetic field in our bodies, we must understand how the meridians work.

What are meridians?

In our bodies, there are numerous "pathways" that convey nervous messages (neurotransmitters). Similarly, blood flows through our arteries, veins, and capillaries, conveying particles of food. Just as there are blood and nerve pathways throughout our bodies, there are other pathways that convey energy. These pathways are the meridians. They can be described as a similar system to the nervous system, but more "delicate" and less tangible.

At this point, we must repeat and clarify a point that is essential for continued reading and understanding, and that will be elaborated upon later. Every organism in the universe, and the universe itself, consists of many different layers, some of them "thicker," that is, more tangible or substantial, and perceivable to the physical senses, and some of them "thinner," more delicate, and not always visible to or perceived by our "regular" senses.

The meridians are a more delicate parallel of the body's

flow systems, while the circulatory system is more tangible, and it is possible to see its vessels and feel it physically, and the nervous system is finer and more delicate, so that we need a microscope to discern its smaller and finer parts, and an electron microscope to see the particles that flow in it, such as neurotransmitters. Although the meridian system is even finer and more delicate, instruments that will enable us to discern it are being developed today.

The meridian system consists of numerous pathways that run the length and breadth of the body, and, like the nervous system, in which there are major nerve centers, there are also meridian points that constitute energetic centers where the paths intersect, and larger energy centers (chakras) that are central energy "gates." According to Chinese medicine, there are innumerable meridians and pathways, but only 26 of them are major (a dozen pairs that appear on the two sides of the body, and two single meridians). Life energy, or chi, flows through the meridians, and from there to the spinal cord and nerves, and to thousands of minor pathways that convey a certain amount of energy.

The spinal cord is considered to be the main axis for the electro-magnetic energy. The north "pole" of human energy is located at the base of the skull (just before the beginning of the first vertebrae in the neck), and the south "pole" is located at the tip of the spinal column. Since the energy pathways flow parallel to one another, there exists among them an interrelated system by means of which they reinforce and stimulate one another. This amplifies the strength of the electro-magnetic field.

In order to safeguard this process of mutual reinforcement and stimulation, the energy currents must be in a normal and harmonious state. To understand the creation of the harmonious or disharmonious state, we must take into account the factors that we have already mentioned - the importance of the state of harmony between our body, mind, and spirit, and the constant energetic relationship between us and our environment and nature, and between us and the universal force. Ultimately, most people who engage in conscious spiritual' activity achieve a profound and intuitive understanding about the existence of the "Supreme Force." At the moment of linking up and genuine, profound introspection, it is possible to feel the energies that are outside of us, or higher energies, being added to our life energy, chi, and in fact joining it and uniting with it. We ourselves are creatures of energy, of light, and the energy system described above is activated in fact by the person's awareness, just like we activate our sensations and thoughts.

The energetic system links our body, mind, and spirit, and is, as mentioned previously, activated by the person's life energy, which controls and understands his life with the help of and through his awareness. When we are in a state of spiritual harmony with the universe, we achieve a harmonious flow in body, mind, and spirit, and our electro-magnetic field expands accordingly.

It would seem that the situation described above leads to the famous paradox, "All is foreseen, but freedom of choice is given" - that is, we are the ones that control our lives, our fate, our happiness, or our suffering, while at the same time, an "invisible" hand directs and leads us. The understanding of the bodies of the aura will take us a step forward toward the apparent understanding (there is no limit to the depth of these matters) of "our" part in this paradox.

The bodies

Many ancient civilizations attest to the fact that there are five bodies, or levels of awareness, that surround the physical body. These are the five bodies, or layers, of the aura. In other civilizations, as well as according to what healers say, various shamans and clairvoyants (people who are blessed with extrasensory perception) count six or seven bodies. For our part, we will concentrate on the five better known and recognized bodies, and will mention the sixth one in a few words. The magnetic and electrical flow of these five bodies of awareness is what creates the outline of the human aura.

The human aura is the energy field that contains all of our knowledge, our past, our present, and our future.

According to the example to which we related in the description of the nature of the meridians, the bodies are also the manifestation of the different things that exist in the universe. As we mentioned previously, there are "coarser," or more "physical," layers that are easily discernible by means of the physical senses, and there are "finer" and more delicate layers. Even people who find it hard to believe in the existence of what the eye can't see (despite the fact that today, thanks to scientific discoveries and the invention of the electron microscope and other similar technical aids, getting "stuck" in the thought pattern that maintains that what we cannot see or touch does not exist, is complete illogical, since we already know that things we cannot see or touch *do* exist, whether we like it or not...) admit that they can often sense the person standing behind them, or next to them, even though he is not touching them; they feel a kind of contact.

This phenomenon stems from the fact that contact

between the bodies of the human being that are further from and broader than the outline of the physical body can be created. (These bodies, as we said before, constitute the aura.) The five bodies of the aura are in a constant state of interaction, and influence one another, as well as the person's sensations, feelings, way of thinking, behavior, and health as a whole. Accordingly, a state of imbalance in one of the bodies will lead to a state of imbalance in other bodies.

The bodies of the aura are as follows:

The first body is the **physical body**, which operates on the given physical planes, that is, it is the "thickest" or most tangible of all the bodies. Our physical body consists of matter - atoms, cells, and organs. It is activated by various biochemical processes, and works according to the laws of time and space, in a physical world, a world of matter. Having said that, in order to understand how much the physical body is affected by the activity and condition of the rest of the bodies, we must relate to the fact that our body consists of atoms, which used to be considered stable, fixed and invariable, until the discovery of quantum physics. As a result, astonishing discoveries were revealed to us: the atom, which had hitherto been considered a particle with a clear, fixed structure, showed itself to be "two-faced." Sometimes it behaves like a particle, and sometimes like a wave! This amazing discovery signifies that we are not just physical and stable, but also energetic, meaning that we live in two worlds simultaneously.

The second body is the **etheric layer (aura)**, which is also called the **aura of the body**. The channels of the meridians are located in this layer. These channels convey life force (chi), and are linked to the body's nervous system. They convey energies and charge the body's energies. The etheric layer is also the one in which diseases begin their path toward physical manifestation, and through it, physical conditions can be treated, because the etheric body is a delicate bio-field that penetrates all matter. This delicate body is responsible for general health and for the person's varied activities. His physical body is fed, develops, and forms under the influence of this delicate energy field.

Although the etheric body is invisible to the human eye, it consists of matter that belongs to the physical world. It is invisible because it vibrates at a higher level than matter does. We often absorb and perceive it unconsciously.

Various mystics and researchers have experienced seeing auras. They describe the aura's matter as misty, located at between one and four inches around the body.

The etheric body channels feelings that affect all the other layers, including the physical body.

The third body is the **emotional layer (aura)**, which is also called the **astral aura**. This layer is connected to our feelings, and affects and is affected by states of emotional imbalance. We can easily understand the activity and the significance of this body when we recall or bring to our mind's eye the state of a person who is angry, nervous, or very upset. Many people who are blessed with reasonable to high sensitivity will feel disturbed and bothered by this person's mass of emotions, even if he does not express them, or does not express them in a hurtful way. People who are more sensitive can sense a stressed, angry, or upset person, even if they meet him by chance in the street, and even if he does everything in his power to hide his emotions. The emotions we feel are manifested in this layer of the aura - in our emotional body.

We cannot discern imbalances in this body in the same way as we can in the physical body (for example, a limp, a cough, and so on), but we can certainly sense them. In fact, the emotional body exists and is tangible just like the physical body, and when a person is nervous, for instance, it is possible to sense the imbalance in his emotional body. Healers or clairvoyants who can discern the emotional aura are likely to be able to discern this imbalance exactly like most of us can discern a physical imbalance, because a state of imbalance in this aura - which is located at a distance of 12 to 16 inches from the physical body - is manifested in the color or shape of the aura. In any event, most people, even if they do not see this aura, can feel its state, and sometimes even be influenced by the state of the emotional aura of someone else.

The fourth body is the **thought layer (aura)**, which is also called the **mental aura**. This layer contains and is affected by our thought patterns and our mental beliefs. When we stick to a particular belief in our thoughts, this is expressed in the aura, which attracts situations that are suitable to our thought pattern. Simply put, the belief or the thought pattern, "I am surrounded by friendly and pleasant people," will attract people of exactly that kind to us by means of its expression in the mental body.

This might all sound a bit simplistic or even unbelievable. However, various experiments that have been performed on the influence of human thought patterns on a person's way of life, as well as on things that were thought, apparently, not to depend on him (for instance, in the workplace - a "nice boss" or an "awful boss," and so on) have shown that many situations in a person's life have been changed drastically by working intensively toward changing thought patterns. Often, working on the subconscious using autosuggestion, hypnosis, and so on, operates on this body. (Not always, however. Sometimes the work is done on the path that joins up with the emotional aura.)

There is a rather blunt saying: "Our thoughts create our reality," or, in an older version from the Kabbalah, "First think, then act."

In other words, physical embodiment, in the world of matter, starts with thought. After thought, speech should occur, followed by action, but thought comes first. Even things that we ostensibly do "without thinking" stem from thought, because our thoughts are not just the conscious thoughts that go through our mind consciously and voluntarily, but are also inner beliefs and conscious or unconscious thought patterns that direct our actions.

The fifth body is the **intuitive layer (aura)**. This layer represents the stratum that is beyond everything that is defined as "knowledge," "logic," and "common sense." Through this layer, we experience "gut feelings," and receive messages, insights, and intuitive information. When this aura layer is "developed," or well balanced, it enables us to experience extrasensory vision and understanding, and it affects and is affected by various types of dreams, telepathic messages, and premonitions. People frequently sense its influence when they get a kind of inexplicable feeling about something that later turns out to be correct, or experience various telepathic situations.

The more balanced this body is, and the person acknowledges and is aware of its presence, the easier it is for the person to receive and decipher the intuitive messages that we actually receive all the time, but are often unaware of them. (We may be aware of them, but we act against them all the same.)

The sixth body is the **karmic-causal layer (aura)**. This aura contains the knowledge concerning our vocation, the reason for our presence in the world in our particular physical body, at the given place and time.

The first aura is the closest to our physical body, and the last is the furthest away from it. Every one of those bodies can be identified by looking at auras, or by sensing auras in various ways.

However, this requires innate ability, or unwavering belief, and a high level of awareness.

Below is a basic exercise for developing awareness and understanding of the various bodies:

Lie or sit comfortably, keeping your spinal column straight.

See that your body is relaxed and calm. Take comfortable abdominal breaths, deep and slow, and let your body release itself and relax while exhaling.

Begin to touch and feel your physical body. Touch your feet, feel your belly, pass your hands over your face, your chest, your knees. Feel your bones, the touch of your skin, your muscles.

In your mind's eye, go in deeper, and visualize yourself feeling your internal organs, which operate so harmoniously in your body.

With the force of your imagination, try to go in even deeper; with your mind's eye, see the cells and atoms of which you are made.

Give yourself time to feel and see your physical body in all its component parts.

Now link up with another part of yourself - your emotions. They are not visible like your physical body and organs, but it is possible to feel them in exactly the same way. Feel your emotions, and the emotional energy that is in you now. What is the emotion that you are feeling? What is the sensation?

In your imagination, recall an annoying incident that occurred recently. Imagine it happening in front of your eyes in every detail. How do you feel? What are the feelings that are going through you? Link up with your physical body for a moment. How does your physical body feel when you imagine the annoying incident? Do you feel any changes in your blood flow or in your muscle tension?

Let the incident go; imagine it being cast into a distant sea, or any place outside of you. Calm down, and relax your body.

Now recall in your mind's eye a happy, moving, or exciting incident that happened recently. Imagine every detail: the characters, the smells, the sounds, and the feelings you felt during those happy moments. Look inside. How do you feel? What are the feelings you are experiencing inside? What kind of emotional energy is going through you?

Link up with your physical body and feel how it takes the incident. Do you feel a broadening in the region of the heart or the abdomen? Are the muscles of your mouth stretching upward?

Inhale deeply and relax your body. You might feel a sensation of might in your belly, power and action.

Take a deep breath into your heart, feel how it opens, feel the tremendous love that is inside you, and let it flow and fill your entire being. These feelings, although you cannot touch them physically, exist inside you and around you all the time.

Now, close your eyes, and focus your attention on what's happening inside your head. Thoughts are passing there; listen to them. What thoughts are going through your head? Listen to them as they pass through your head. Pay attention to how they pass. You can listen to your thoughts.

"Catch" one of the thoughts, and change it into any other form. You are able to examine your thoughts. If so, you are not your thoughts. You are a witness to them. You activate them. You can direct them. They do not control you. You can control them and direct them at will.

Try and remain in this state of awareness for a few minutes. In this state, you feel and are aware of and alert to your various bodies; you notice that they are part of you, and that you have the ability to get involved in, control, and watch their activities.

Practicing this exercise from time to time will help you to achieve a higher state of awareness about your aura layers, to internalize your ability to control them, and to take full responsibility for them.

Since the auras are closely interrelated, and a state of imbalance in one of the bodies affects the others. As a result, practically speaking, there is no such thing as a purely "physical disease" or a purely "mental disease," and so on. When a person succumbs to a physical disease, or any other kind of disease, if we look at him carefully, we can find an imbalance in the other layers (that in most cases is the same kind of imbalance that manifested itself physically).

As an example, we will describe the development of a very common problem that is considered "easy" to describe from the point of view of embodying the different layers. Constipation is a problem suffered by many in the modern world. It is manifested in an obvious way in the physical body, and is liable to lead to many complications, such as excessive toxins in the digestive tract, a bloated feeling, chronically impaired digestion, and so on. When we wish to examine the source of the constipation in the emotional-mental layer, we sometimes discover that it lies in the inability to let go (which is actually what happens in physical constipation!). It could be that if we look at the person's traits, we will find that he finds it difficult to let go of things - money, old, unwanted property, incidents from his past, and so on. When we examine his emotional-sentimental behavior, we may see that he finds it difficult to release emotions as well; he stops himself from expressing love, anger, or any other emotion, or finds it hard to let certain people go, and so on. If we look at his mental, or thought behavior, we may find that he clings to old thought patterns that he "inherited" from his parents or other factors, and refuses to release them, even though logically speaking there is no point in holding on to them. This clinging to unnecessary old thought patterns may manifest itself in the intuitive level as an inability to receive information and new insights, to be open to different messages, or to heed his gut feelings, and in this way, his intuitive abilities are impaired.

Of course, this is only an example, and every person should be related to individually, weighing up the sum of his problems against the qualities of his personality and his body - but it shows the interrelationship between our various bodies.

The influences of the karmic layer or aura are extremely important, but very few people know how to identify and understand them. If they do, it is usually by means of channeling abilities, receiving messages from superior forces, or the ability to discern from the person's previous incarnations which lesson he has to learn in his present incarnation in this world. Karmic influences can be some kind of handicap, for example, birth defects, cruel acts or crimes perpetrated against the person, serious mental diseases, perpetual poverty, and so on. Having said that, we must remember the saying, "All is foreseen, but freedom of choice is given," that is, even with the various kinds of karmic influences, the person can and must cope by balancing all his bodies, and the karmic influences exist to teach him how to deal with a certain situation in the purest and most correct way.

The problems, or the imbalance, are ostensibly liable to begin in any one of the bodies, but it is not easy to distinguish which one preceded which - "the chicken or the egg" - if this kind of "precedence" exists at all. The reason for this, as we stated earlier, is the extremely close interrelationship among the bodies.

All of these problems or states of imbalance and disharmony are indicative of blockages in the person's bodies. Just as the blood flow, for example, needs healthy and pliant arteries and veins in order to flow normally, so the energy flow requires open and healthy channels, devoid of blockages. The correct, natural, and smooth flow of energy will lead to equilibrium in every layer, and will of course afford the person physical, mental, and spiritual health.

Free passages of energy are important and significant. When these passages are balanced, the person's ability to absorb and receive energy (which is influenced by the equilibrium and harmony of the bodies) is also balanced. When we examine the sophisticated way in which we are constructed, physically and energetically - so that we can be "vessels" or energetic "transmitters" to the life energy, or chi - the question arises as to the source of this energy that activates, influences, and realizes our being.

In the past, various philosophers tended to think - mainly on the basis of theoretical formulas - that the nature of energy was inside the person, and that the person in fact constituted a "closed circuit" from the energetic point of view that nourished and balanced itself by means of his self-energy. In contrast, many civilizations, religions, and thinkers believe that the source of energy is in a tremendous energetic force that is found everywhere, always, and in everything. Some called this force "God," "the Great Spirit," "universal force," and other names, including attributing the receiving of energy to nature (which, too, is the embodiment of the universal force, or God, of course). Whatever it is called, it gives man life, and influences his movement, just as it influences the movement of the stars, the spinning of the earth on its axis, or the movement of atomic particles. This prodigious energy "seeps" into the person's being. The very fact of the energy being in him makes the person "godlike" too, in a certain sense.

This opinion, which is based mainly on spiritual experiences, as well as on scientific discoveries, is the most accepted one amongst people who deal with, see, or feel energy. The reason for this is very simple: examining the aura. When a person develops this ability, he can see how, in various situations the person whose aura he is examining receives a "surge" of energy, in a certain form, from an external source. For example, it is sometimes possible to see that when the person performs meditation for linking up, or prayer, there is a line, a circle or circles, or a cone of light above his head, and they link up to him.

I remember looking at the aura of a master guitarist who was improvising a melody on his guitar - something he was composing as he went along. The sight of the inverted cone of white light like a kind of funnel above his head gave tangible and very comprehensible meaning to the term "artist par excellence." When music is pure, and free of ego, it is an old and well-known form of divine channeling, just like prayer or meditation.

In order to receive this energy, the person must be clean and pure (spiritually, and preferably also physically), feel a desire to receive it, and be eligible to receive it. In principle, the person is supposed to - and deserves to - receive exactly the "helping" of energy that is appropriate for him at a given moment of his physical, mental, and spiritual development. Sometimes people try to draw a larger quantity of this energy, either by so-called material means of "amassing" or "hoarding" energy, or by attempts to draw more of the energy in its pure, or more spiritual form. Drawing too large a quantity of energy by artificial means (such as drugs, for instance), is liable to lead to a situation in which the person cannot contain the amount of energy, and the result could be negative, even dangerous - exactly like not receiving a sufficient amount of energy is liable to manifest itself in various states of imbalance, such as fatigue, weakness, lack of vitality, and so on.

How is this energy channeled into our body in a correct and harmonious form, and how do the energetic passage and the link between the various bodies occur? The answer to these questions can be found by understanding the action of the chakras.

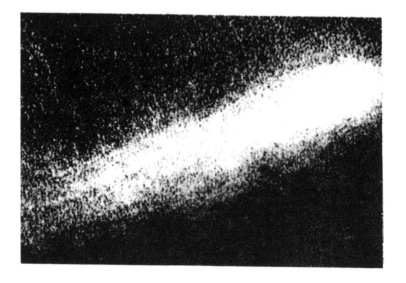

The chakras

Many ancient civilizations relate to energy centers through which energy passes, entering and leaving and changing the body's energy field. According to the Hopi tribe in North America, the human body is built according to the same principles as the earth. Both the earth and human beings have an axis. The earth's north-south polar axis parallels the spinal column, the north pole parallels the brain, and the south pole parallels the base of the spinal column - the coccyx. The spinal column is responsible for the body's balance. Not only are the nerve centers located along this axis, but so are the energy centers. The centers are responsible for the person's physical, mental, and spiritual functioning.

Oriental medicine relates in depth to the significance of the etheric body and the energy centers in human beings. The Indians call these centers "chakras." The word "chakra" means "wheel." Every chakra manifests itself in the physical body, mainly in one of the endocrine glands that regulate all the physical and mental processes of the human body. Higher - cosmic - energies are channeled through the chakras to the physical and other human bodies. This energy, which is also called life energy, flows through the chakras, and is of cardinal importance for our lives and for our physical, mental, and spiritual health. When a situation arises in which the energy does not flow through the chakras in a harmonious manner, or when one of the chakras is either blocked or open too wide, an imbalance occurs, and this is evident in every aspect of life. The state of imbalance in the chakra will affect the endocrine gland to which the chakra is linked, and the body's delicate metabolic balance will be upset.

Each of the aura layers mentioned in the previous chapter, in addition to the material body - as well as everything else that exists in the universe - has its own unique vibrational frequency. In human beings, all the aura layers are supposed to be harmoniously joined and linked. If one of the aura layers is not linked to the others, the passage of information and energy between the bodies is disrupted.

For instance, when there is a rift between the mental (thought) body and the emotional body, a situation in which the person is unable to express his thoughts is liable to occur. Another rift causes a situation in which the person is unable to translate his emotions and thoughts into creation or action; and so on.

Like every other sophisticated "appliance" that works according to the principle of giving and taking (receiving and transmitting), human beings also require centers for receiving, transmitting, and converting of energy. These centers are the chakras. In the physical body, the chakras function as "transmitters." They transmit the currents that arrive from the higher, more refined energy, which operates on higher frequencies of energetic bodies, to the physical body, while "converting" the frequency to a frequency that our physical body can use.

In the same way that domestic use of electrical energy at a different frequency can cause a short-circuit, so it is if the energy that operates at higher frequencies is not converted in human beings. We can compare the action of the human body to the way in which we use electricity. We get our electrical energy from a source that contains enormously powerful electricity (the Electric Company). Electrical energy is conveyed to private homes by means of cables that carry electricity in appropriate and correct quantities, and not more. If too powerful an electric current were to be conveyed to a home, the results would be disastrous. On the other hand, plants and factories that require a large amount of electricity, and have a suitable infrastructure, receive and consume a much larger amount of electricity than private homes.

The aura layer that absorbs and contains the person's breath of life within it is the spiritual body, which is our divine side, and links us to creation. From this link, the energy passes to the other aura layers, each of which has a different purpose and vocation, and for that reason, requires a different quality of energy at a different frequency.

On each level, there are stations that convert the energy into a form that is suitable for the next level.

The entire universe is linked by a tremendous, primeval force. This force is transferred to every thing and every creature, according to their capacity, and in accordance with the frequencies that are compatible with them from the physiological, emotion, intellectual, and spiritual points of view. When the energy makes its way from this tremendous, primeval force to the bodies in the universe, its power and strength seem to decrease more and more, so that these bodies can absorb it, since they cannot cope with even one particle of the "non-decreased" power.

The human body, like the universe, consists of different strata - a spiritual stratum, an emotional stratum, and an intellectual stratum. The difference between the human body and the "body" of the cosmos lies solely in their wavelengths and frequencies. For that reason, the divine force is found not only outside of us, but also inside us. Since human beings have the ability to use the gift of the imagination, they can tune themselves intellectually, intuitively, or emotionally to the various energy bodies and strata of awareness, and change them.

Every method that broadens awareness, such as positive thinking, directed imagining, meditation, and many others, helps people tune themselves.

The chakras and awareness

Our awareness is our strongest tool as human beings. Our awareness can move about in our multidimensional being via the different strata. These changes - which are, in fact, the movement - may occur regularly and quickly. For this reason, the energy centers of the body are extremely important. Every chakra serves as a relay and transmitting station to a particular zone of frequency or awareness. When attention is focused on one of the chakras, the person is consciously or unconsciously involved mainly with the areas for which that chakra is "responsible."

With the help of their spiritual abilities, the sages of ancient China and India received information about the human energy system. They wrote this information down in vedas, which contain the ancient knowledge.

In India, as in other ancient and enlightened civilizations, the chakras are linked to particular colors, elements, symbols, and characteristics. The combination of these factors, which are linked to a certain chakra - for instance, during the chanting of a mantra that is attributed to that chakra, while looking at a certain shape of a certain color - creates a certain frequency that may link up, at a certain resonance, to a certain element in the human body. For example, the earth element is linked to the sex glands, to the first chakra, to the planet Mars, to the color red, to the ruby... and so on. This technique affords general equilibrium, which affects the person as well as the factors that are involved in the process.

This action also works in the opposite direction. When the person concentrates on a certain characteristic, wish, or ambition, allows them to dominate his life, and lives according to them, a situation is created whereby he works, lives and communicates more from within the chakra that is linked to the area to which he attributes extreme importance. This is again a situation of "What came first - the chicken or the egg?" in which a certain perception, way of thinking, and form of behavior lead to an imbalance in the chakras. This imbalance is liable to exacerbate the situation enormously. It is difficult to say whether the imbalance in the chakras is what caused the behavioral, thought, and emotional imbalance, or vice versa.

Let's take a look at a common example of this imbalance. A person's sole interest is in increasing his income, and amassing more and more money and property. He spends most of his time concentrating on mundane problems and material and physical matters, and pays no attention to intellectual, mental, or spiritual development at a higher level. This person's awareness is focused significantly on the first chakra, and most of his thoughts concern survival, income, and material issues. But even when most of the person's focus of interest is linked to a particular chakra - in an unbalanced manner - it is liable to manifest itself in a number of ways. For example, excessive concentration on the first chakra may characterize a person with violent impulses, and a lust for mammon or sex - or, on the other hand, this strong energy may be characterized by a powerful life force and a high degree of vitality. So, even concentration on a particular chakra - which ultimately creates some kind of imbalance - is likely to be expressed in many different forms, according to the development of the individual personality.

In the same way, the chakra's colors, as they are manifested in the aura, may also change. In the above example, the color of the first, or base, chakra, may appear in different shades of red, ranging from dark, "dirty" red, which indicates extreme materialistic behavior, or even addiction to drugs or alcohol, to light, "clean" red, which may attest to a sensitive person who copes with his surroundings well, but is also very interested in material matters. This situation may occur in the other chakras, and, of course, will be expressed in the colors of the entire aura.

The more a person concentrates and focuses on one area of life and awareness - such as creativity, materialism, mental development, spiritual development, and so on - the more obvious this fact will be in the action of the chakra that is responsible for this area. Because of the interrelationship among the chakras, it affects the state of the other chakras, all the person's realms of awareness and being, and his aura layers.

When a strong frequency of a particular color - yellow, for instance - is seen in the aura, it means that most of the person's awareness is concentrated on the "yellow" chakra - the third or solar plexus chakra. This may be an indication of a sensitive stomach, and a situation in which the third chakra is open or opens at the time. On the other hand, this can indicate a greater amount of concentration on the action of the third chakra - for example, the desire to be freer, or totally independent. These desires, which lead to focusing on the action of the third chakra, radiate onto the entire aura, and turn the yellow into the dominant color at that time.

The aura layers are linked to the aura, to the electro-magnetic field, by means of the chakras.

According to the colors of the person's aura, it is possible to know if his awareness is based more in the physical, mental, spiritual, or intellectual stratum, and if there is a certain imbalance between these areas and the action of the chakras.

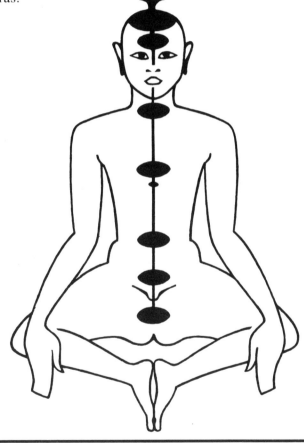

The significance of the chakras

As we explained earlier, every chakra is linked to a particular color, sense, sound, element, endocrine gland, symbol, crystal, and body, as well as certain physical, mental, and spiritual characteristics.

There are numerous energy centers - like chakras - in the human body. In various ancient systems, more than seven major chakras are described. (In the Kabbalah, for instance, the "spheres," of which there are ten, parallel the chakras; in certain Oriental systems, 13 centers are mentioned; and so on.) However, here we will focus on the seven major chakras that are the best known and the most widely accepted.

The first chakra - the Base (Root) Chakra

This chakra symbolizes the struggle to survive, the basic needs, the ability to be assertive, and the link to the earth. It is also called the Root Chakra, and its Indian name is **Muladhara**, which means "base" or "root." The chakra is located between the anus and the genitals. Its colors are black and red. (Black does not appear in the aura's colors, but it is possible to balance the chakra by means of certain black stones, and therefore black is also one of its colors.) According to ancient Indian writings, the sense that is linked to this chakra is the sense of smell, and the sound that is linked to it, according to those writings, is "lam."

In the Indian tradition, the sign or symbol that relates to this chakra is a circle surrounded by four lotus leaves, with a square inside it, sometimes in yellow-gold, symbolizing the material world, and containing the letters of the sound "lam." A kind of "pipe" emerges from it, symbolizing the link of the chakra to the rest of the chakras and to the universal force that fills it with energy. The element that is linked to this chakra is earth, and the endocrine glands that are linked to it are the sex glands.

The organs linked to this chakra are the spinal column and the skeleton, the excretory organs, and the reproductive and physical continuity organs.

This chakra is linked to the person's basic survival instinct, to existential fears, to his ability to be practical and to function successfully in the material world, to the ability to have both feet firmly on the ground, and to make decisions. It links spiritual ability and the physical expression of this ability. When the chakra is in a state of harmonious action, it is expressed in powerful sexuality, being energetic and active, strong vitality, stability, and the ability to discern. An imbalance in the chakra is expressed in sexual promiscuity, sexual imbalance, deep anxiety, aggressiveness, disproportional focus on money and material things, lust for sex and mammon, lack of confidence, instability, detachment, delusion, and strong egocentricity.

From the physical point of view, an imbalance in this chakra is liable to be expressed in infertility, venereal diseases or diseases associated with sexuality, hemorrhoids, constipation, and problems in the skeleton and joints.

The stones that are used for treating and balancing this chakra are red and black ones, among them ruby, snowflake obsidian, black tourmaline, smoky quartz (whose color actually tends to gray; it is also used for the crown chakra, and links the upper chakras to the lower ones), and dark bloodstone.

The second chakra - the Sex Chakra

This chakra symbolizes emotions, sexuality, and sensuality. Its Indian name is **Svadhisthana**, which means "inside the body." The chakra is located on the pelvis, between the pubic bones. Its color is mainly orange, but also yellow that tends to orange. According to ancient Indian writings, the sense that is linked to this chakra is the sense of taste, and the sound that is linked to it, according to those writings, is "vam."

The sign that relates to this chakra is a circle surrounded by five lotus leaves, with a circle inside it (usually red), symbolizing and containing the letters of the sound "vam." A kind of "pipe" emerges from it, symbolizing the link of the chakra to the rest of the chakras and to the universal force. Sometimes a silver-gray crescent appears inside the circle. The element that is linked to this chakra is water, and the endocrine gland that is linked to it is the adrenal gland.

The organs linked to this chakra are the blood and the lymph, the digestive juices, the kidneys, the bladder, the muscles, and the sex organs.

This chakra symbolizes change and individuality, while understanding the uniqueness of other people. It is linked to enjoyment, sexuality, the desire to procreate, self-satisfaction, creativity, self-realization, and devotion to one's personal path. When the chakra is not balanced, this is expressed in many unrequited passions, which the person tries to realize in all kinds of ways (such as addiction to sex or food, and so on), a tendency to be jealous, restlessness, a lack of sexual balance, and problems in creating social and conjugal ties (problems that lead to loneliness).

From the physical point of view, a state of disharmony in

the chakra is expressed in unbalanced circulation, kidney and gallbladder problems, frigidity, impotence, and muscular problems.

The stones that are used for treating and balancing this chakra are orange ones, or orange with a reddish tendency, such as amber, coral, blood-opal, garnet, and ruby.

The third chakra - the Solar Plexus Chakra

This chakra symbolizes the development of the personality, the ability to influence, power, and the practical facet of the intellect. The Indian name of this chakra is **Manipura**, which means "the palace of the diamond." The chakra is located on the solar plexus, in the region of the diaphragm. Its color is mainly yellow, but also blue. According to ancient Indian writings, the sense that is linked to this chakra is the sense of sight, and the sound that is linked to it, according to Indian tradition, is "ram."

The sign that relates to this chakra is a circle surrounded by ten lotus leaves, with a triangle inside it (usually red), containing the letters of the sound "ram." A kind of "pipe" emerges from it, symbolizing the link of the chakra to the rest of the chakras and to the universal force. The element that is linked to this chakra is fire, and the endocrine gland that is linked to it is the pancreas.

The organs linked to this chakra are the respiratory system and the diaphragm, the digestive system, the stomach, the pancreas, the liver, the spleen, the gallbladder, the small intestine, the extra-renal glands, and the sympathetic nervous system.

This chakra represents the ego; it is the source of all feelings and emotions, deeds, strength, self-will, the I, and realizing the I. Through this chakra, the person links up to the outside world and interprets it according to the balance of the chakra. When the chakra is in a state of balance, the person is courageous, creative, independent, tolerant, and strong in personality. An imbalance in the chakra is expressed in an unbalanced ego, dependence, manipulative behavior, exploitation of power, domineering behavior, arrogance, and fears.

From the physical point of view, an imbalance in this chakra is expressed in the physical body as problems in the liver, the gallbladder, and the eyes.

The stones that are used for treating and balancing this chakra are stones in all shades of yellow, such as citrine, amber, yellow topaz, yellow malachite, and so on.

The fourth chakra - the Heart Chakra

This chakra symbolizes love, caring, devotion, the ability to cure and heal, giving, and a lack of selfishness. Its Indian name is **Anahata**, which means "the ever-beating drum." The chakra is located in the center of the chest, parallel to the heart, and it links the upper chakras to the lower ones. Its colors are pink and green. According to Indian tradition, the sense that is linked to this chakra is the sense of touch, and the sound that is linked to it, according to ancient Indian writings, is "yam."

The sign or symbol that relates to this chakra is a circle surrounded by twelve lotus leaves, with a six-pointed star inside it, containing the letters of the sound "yam." A kind of "pipe" emerges from it, symbolizing the link of the chakra to the rest of the chakras and to the universal force. An additional symbolic element associated with this chakra is gray-green smoke. The element that is linked to this chakra is air, and the endocrine gland that is linked to it is the thymus gland.

The organs linked to this chakra are the heart, the circulatory system, the lungs, the immune system, the thymus gland, the skin, and the hands.

This chakra is linked to the ability to love, the ability to give and receive love unconditionally, forgiveness, compassion, generosity of heart and pocket, unselfishness, and the will and ability to give to others. It links spiritual ability and the physical expression of this ability. If the chakra is in a state of disharmony, it is expressed in selfishness, an inability to give and receive love, fears and anxieties, lust for mammon, stinginess, hesitancy, and indecisiveness.

Because this chakra links the lower chakras with the upper ones, when this chakra is blocked, the effects of the blockage are felt in the entire body.

From the physical point of view, an imbalance in this chakra is liable to be expressed in asthma, and circulatory, respiratory, and cardiac problems.

The stones that are used for treating and balancing this chakra are green and pink ones, such as rose quartz, green tourmaline, pink tourmaline, rhodochrosite, opal, kunzite, and so on.

The fifth chakra - the Throat Chakra

This chakra symbolizes creativity, the ability to express oneself, communication, and inspiration. Its Indian name is **Visuddha**, which means "full of purity." The chakra is located in the throat. Its colors are blue and light-blue. According to Indian tradition, the sense that is linked to this chakra is the sense of hearing.

The sign that relates to this chakra is a circle surrounded by sixteen lotus leaves, with a circle inside it, or a circle with a triangle inside it. A kind of "pipe" emerges from it, containing the letters of the sound "ham." The element that is linked to this chakra is blue sky, and the endocrine gland that is linked to it is the thyroid gland.

The organs linked to this chakra are the throat, the neck, the vocal cords, the vocal organs, the thyroid gland, the nerves, the ears, and the muscles.

This chakra is linked to all aspects of communication, the ability to communicate well, harmony with one's surroundings, the ability to express oneself, creativity, self-image, and faith. It links thought to the expression of thought. If the chakra is in a state of disharmony, it is expressed in communication problems, the inability to express thoughts and desires, a lack of creativity, anger, apathy, indifference, and conflicts between emotion and logic.

From the physical point of view, an imbalance in this chakra is expressed in inflammations, infections, and vocal problems.

The stones that are used for treating and balancing this chakra are stones in shades of blue, light-blue, and turquoise, such as blue lace agate, aquamarine, topaz, lapis lazuli, blue sapphire, chrysocolla, amazonite, celestite, sodalite, and gem-silica.

The sixth chakra - the Third Eye Chakra

This chakra symbolizes intuition, intellectual power, will power, and knowledge. Its Indian name is **Ajna**, which means "command center." The chakra is located on the forehead, between the eyebrows. Its colors are purple and indigo. According to Indian tradition, the sense that is linked to this chakra is the intuition (the sixth sense), and the sound that is linked to it is "kasham."

The sign that relates to this chakra is a sky-blue circle surrounded on both sides by large lotus leaves, with a drawing of two feet inside it. A kind of "pipe" emerges from it, containing the letters of the sound "kasham." The element that is linked to this chakra is ether, and the endocrine gland that is linked to it is the pituitary gland, which is responsible for the action of all the endocrine glands and all hormonal action.

The organs linked to this chakra are the various parts of the brain, the central nervous system, the face, the eyes, the ears, and the nose.

This chakra is the one that links the person to his subconscious, intuition, the ability to comprehend cosmic insights and to receive non-verbal messages. It is responsible for balancing the two cerebral hemispheres, left and right, that is, intuition and emotion (and mysticism) with logic and reason. It is also responsible for physical balance, the ability to concentrate, peace of mind, wisdom, and extra-sensory perception. When the chakra is balanced, the person will have the qualities of popularity, powerful intuition, high morality, and clarity. If the chakra is in a state of imbalance, it is expressed in depression, dependence, unrequited passions, indecisiveness, imbalance, mental exhaustion, auditory and visual problems, and learning and comprehension problems.

From the physical point of view, an imbalance in this chakra is liable to be expressed in headaches, nightmares, nerve problems, and ear and eye problems.

The stones that are used for treating and balancing this chakra are ones that are purple and indigo, such as amethyst, sodalite, lapis lazuli, azurite, sugilite, and fluorite.

The seventh chakra - the Crown Chakra

This chakra symbolizes enlightenment, knowledge, and linking up to the higher strata of spiritual awareness. Its Indian name is **Sasharata**, which means "the lotus flower with a thousand petals." The chakra is located on the crown of the head. Its colors are purple and white. The sense that is linked to this chakra is the finest and most delicate sense that constitutes the ability to tune oneself in to supreme messages and the universal force (which perhaps can be called "the sense of enlightenment"). The sound that is linked to it is "om."

The sign that relates to this chakra is a lotus with a thousand petals with the letters of the sound "om" above it. The element that is linked to this chakra is the ether and space element, and the endocrine gland that is linked to it is the pineal gland.

The organ linked to this chakra is the brain.

This chakra is responsible for linking up to higher

awareness, the ability to receive divine and cosmic insights, and the ability to link up to divine knowledge and the light of universal love. When the chakra is open and balanced, the person is blessed with enlightenment, and enjoy a harmonious and satisfying life. If the chakra is in a state of imbalance, it is liable to be expressed in boredom, a lack of purpose, the inability to open up to spiritual dimensions, the lack of perfect awareness, extreme situations, and situations of coma and death.

The stones that are used for treating and balancing this chakra are mainly purple and white ones, such as clear quartz, pyrite, white jade, white tourmaline, and diamond.

PART 2

COLORS

When the significance and action of the aura and the chakras were investigated in the first part of this book, you no doubt noticed that a place of honor was accorded the color that was linked to each chakra. The link between the color and the particular chakra is neither arbitrary nor a human invention. People who are blessed with the gift of seeing auras, or who have developed this ability - and there are quite a few of them - are in agreement about the colors that each of the chakras transmits!

From personal experience, and acquaintance with many people who can see the colors of the aura and the chakras, I see these links between colors, auras, and chakras as a solid, tangible fact.

It is no coincidence that such a lot of importance is attributed to the color in the context of the aura, or to our physical, mental, or spiritual state.

The aura, the electro-magnetic field that surrounds the human body, is composed of all the colors of the spectrum, with different combinations and emphases. The astral body, for instance, contains an extremely delicate balance of colors, and every state of imbalance will be expressed in the predominance of certain colors among the colors of the aura (or in the weakening or disappearance of certain colors). This balance is essential and significant for the general health of the person, and for every aspect of his life. While the balance is preserved, the person will feel healthy and calm, and his life will be harmonious, free-flowing, and satisfying. When the balance is upset, various diseases, types of discomfort, unbalanced moods, and negative states such as fatigue, nervousness, depression, and so on, are liable to occur. As a result, states of imbalance in various areas of his life - such as his marriage, work, creativity, and so on - occur.

The imbalance between the colors of the aura is liable to be long-term and protracted, or temporary, if it stems form a specific reason, such as following an emotional outburst, a row, a quarrel, or the arrival of bad news. During those painful situations, and after them, too - until the person finally liberates himself from the morass of negative emotions - a situation of imbalance in the colors of the aura is liable to be created, with certain colors becoming very weak. Occasionally, all the colors of the spectrum may become weak, muddy, or faded.

What *is* color?

From the point of view of physics, color is energy with a defined wavelength and frequency. Every color has its own wavelength and frequency. Color energy influences the entire cosmos, and the human organism that is a part of it. Everything in the world, including the human organism, has a particular vibrational frequency, and every vibration has its own frequency. There are many frequencies that human beings are unable to pick up with their ordinary senses, such as X-rays, gamma rays, infra-red light, and so on. Among the many frequencies, there is a relatively small group of frequencies that we can see with our eyes: the colors red, orange, yellow, green, blue, indigo, and purple. These colors each have a different frequency and wavelength. The length of the wave in the range of light that the eye can see ranges between 740 nanometers in the color red, and 400 nanometers in the color purple. The human eye can only pick up the colors within the range of these two wave frequencies. Red light has the longest wave and the shortest vibrational frequency. (Infra-red light, however, is invisible to the human eye.) Purple light has the shortest wave and the highest vibrational frequency. (Ultra-violet light, however is invisible to the human eye.)

Both colors that are visible to the human eye, and those that are not, exert a significant influence on our organism and on our moods. It is a fact that red light, which has the shortest vibrational frequency, is attributed to the lowest chakra - the base (root) chakra. In contrast, purple light has the highest vibrational frequency, and was attributed, long before color wavelengths and frequencies were measured, to the highest chakra of human awareness - the third eye chakra - as well as to the crown chakra above it. This astounding fact is indicative of the extra-sensory abilities of people of the ancient civilizations.

In color therapy, the various frequencies of the visible colors of the spectrum are utilized in order to alter a particular physical or mental state. In healing and medicine, the invisible colors, such as infra-red and ultra-violet, are also utilized. Color therapy first developed when psychological changes caused by the different colors were discerned. Every color sparks different associations, emotions, and feelings in the human brain. It is almost certain that some of the feelings and most of the associations are subjective and personal, and differ from person to person.

However, it is difficult to ignore the fact that there is a certain consensus - possibly even an unconscious one - pertaining to the feelings that each color evokes.

For instance, most people to whom you show the color red will tell you that it evokes an association of warning, war, blood, passion, desire, sexuality, and so on. In contrast, the color green evokes associations of calmness, plant life, peace, and so on in most people

Although we impose our subjective associations on a color when we are relating to it, the energetic "objective" action of the color affects our way of relating to it.

The strong mental effect of colors on our nervous system, on our emotions, on our aura, and possibly also on our hormonal system, has caused many psychologists, therapists, and healers - as well as interior designers, architects, and artists - to utilize colors to evoke numerous feelings in the observer or the patient. When it comes to painting the walls of our homes, we, too, consider the color in relation to the given space, knowing - almost instinctively - that a light color creates a feeling of greater space, while a dark color creates an illusion of less space. Very few people paint the walls of their homes black, both because of the negative connotation attached to this all-devouring color, and because of the unpleasant feeling it evokes in the inhabitants.

In view of all this, it is not surprising that many nervous and mental diseases have been alleviated and even cured following a change in the color of the patient's surroundings, sometimes by transferring him to a room painted in a color that is beneficial for him. The dominant colors in emergency rooms are green and white, colors that are considered to be the optimal general healing colors.

Understanding the extraordinary action of colors on the human organism is not the preserve of progress or the last generation only, but has a historic tradition that stretches back thousands of years.

The history of the use of colors

The use of color for treating diseases, protection, raising one's spirits, attracting a mate, and many more, has been known for thousands of years, encompassing all the members of all the different civilizations.

Even in prehistoric times, colors were used to paint pictures on cave walls and for decorating the body before the hunt or before burial. The warriors of ancient civilizations would anoint their bodies with "war paint," and it is interesting that the same colors - mainly red and white - were used by warriors of different civilizations and on different continents.

The strong effect of color on the human mind, and the ability to use it to express many situations and emotions were manifested in the broad use of it by people from time immemorial for dyeing their clothes, for adorning and painting their houses (to this day, in Arab villages, for example, many houses are decorated with a turquoise-blue stripe, which serves as protection against the evil eye; in many civilizations, the same colors serve the identical purpose), and for attracting a mate (an ancient use that is still very much in evidence today, in the form of make-up).

Using color is not the sole preserve of humans. The plant and animal kingdoms were given the gift of colors by nature, since in these kingdoms the importance of colors is cardinal and fundamental to the continuation of the species and its survival, as we see in numerous examples in the animal world. For instance, certain colors are used as warning colors to chase predators away; as camouflage that enable the animals to move around their territory almost indiscernibly; and as mating colors that help the male, in most species, attract the female for the purpose of mating and perpetuating the species.

The significance of colors is expressed on various levels: on the physical level (as was described in the animal world), on the emotional level, and on the spiritual level.

On the emotional level, it is very easy to feel the influence of color on the human nervous system. Different colors arouse different feelings and emotions. Imagine being in a room that is painted completely black, as opposed to being in a room that is painted in delicate, harmonious colors. The feeling that results from being in each of these rooms is totally different.

In order to understand and feel the effect of color more profoundly, conduct an experiment with yourself: Choose to dress for a day in exactly the colors you don't like, and almost never wear. If you are aware of and tuned into your feelings on that day, and aware of the reactions and behavior of the people around you, you are likely to make amazing discoveries about the effect of color!

As the number of psychological experiments concerning the effect of color on the mind increases, general knowledge about the effect of color is also growing. The fact that a particular color may induce tranquillity or spur people on to action, or bring calmness or cause pressure, is exploited today by psychologists and interior designers alike (as well as by companies and institutions like banks, and even private houses).

In the ancient world, most of the knowledge and understanding of the action of colors belonged to the tribal healers, the holy men, the mystics, and the painters. Today, thanks to scientific research conducted mainly in the fields of physics and psychology to investigate and explain the action of color from the physical point of view, and its effect on the nervous system and on the electro-magnetic field, the use of color therapy is widespread, and the understanding of the nature of color is constantly increasing. Furthermore, those spiritual and mystical contexts that are also expressed in color are becoming the preserve of many more people, because of the spiritual openness and the great amount of "arcane" knowledge that has entered the public domain.

Color is very significant in our daily lives. Our mood is likely to influence our choice of color in clothing, for instance, and a particular color of clothing may affect our mood (as you will no doubt discover, if you do the experiment mentioned previously).

Taking a good look at our attraction to various colors is likely to teach us about our ambitions, our mood, and our general situation. A person who wears a lot of orange may feel a need to increase his self-confidence, his energy level, his vitality and joy; while another person who wears a lot of blue may reveal himself to be a person who aspires to tranquillity and calmness.

Of course, those are fairly superficial examples, but by taking a good look at the color of people's clothes, especially those of acquaintances, you can discover the connections between a choice of color in clothing and the behavior or aspirations of the person.

The significance of colors

As we have already explained, colors exert an enormous influence on the human organism - body, mind, and spirit. In color therapy, in therapies that treat the aura, and in healing - as well as in the traditions of many ancient, enlightened societies - the various colors are linked to various abilities or qualities. Although there are astounding and surprising parallels between insights that originate in various ancient civilizations and the revelations and knowledge of healers, it must be remembered that the significance of every color varies - slightly or greatly - from person to person, according to his "bank of associations," experience, and many other parameters.

Warm colors

All the warm colors - red, orange, and yellow - have arousing and stimulating properties, and are linked to the masculine energy, the yang, as it is known in the Orient.

Red

Red is the color of the base (root) chakra. It symbolizes the element of fire, which is essential for all creatures. Like fire, the color red stimulates, warms, arouses, intensifies vitality, inspires persistence, passion, and ambitiousness. It is used in color therapy for treating conditions of stagnation, and when it is necessary to stimulate life energy or renew it.

The color red is linked to the heart, the circulatory system, the sexual organs, the kidneys, and the bladder. It is used for stimulating the liver, for anemic conditions, for increasing the production of red blood cells, for stimulating the circulatory system, spinal fluid, and the nervous system. It is beneficial for states of exhaustion, arthritis, muscle pains, hernias, bacterial diseases, and impotence. Red is also used for treating diseases of the sensory nerves, such as problems concerning hearing, taste, smell, sight, and touch. Red stimulates slow or inert metabolism, and accelerates the expulsion of toxins and metabolic waste. It helps to relieve constipation, expands the blood vessels, and assists in the production of blood.

Because of the color red's ability to warm and stimulate to a great extent, color therapists and healers tend not to use red on its own, but rather in combination with blue, or with the complementary color of red - turquoise.

The color red is not suitable - either in clothing or in therapy - for people who suffer from being too hot, who are hot-headed or agitated, or who suffer from high blood pressure and flushed faces.

When red appears in the aura in a balanced way, it attests to a great deal of vitality, good physical health, a warm and enthusiastic nature, strength, strong will power, independence, alertness, openness, extroversion, emotionalism, motivation, leadership ability, courage, passion, sexuality and sensuality, and, from the spiritual point of view, "divine fire."

When red appears in the aura in an unbalanced way, it attests to aggressiveness, anger, violence, destructiveness, confusion, frustration, vengefulness, rebelliousness, tyranny, domination, insanity, hyperactivity, tension, and impotence.

Light red attests to sexuality, passion, eroticism, gaiety, femininity, sensitivity, love.

Dark red attests to physical strength, will power, masculinity, leadership ability, courage, rage, yearning, hostility and irascibility.

Dark brown is not considered to be one of the self-standing colors of the aura, but rather a color that appears during a particular situation, which generally indicates an imbalance. Thus, when it does appear among the colors of the aura, it is usually not a good sign. It can attest to egoism, difficulty in giving and receiving love, exaggerated earthiness, various addictions, disease, and destruction.

Orange

Orange is the color of the second chakra, the sex chakra. Orange comprises a mixture of red and yellow. Like red, it is also a warm color, and is thus blessed with the ability to arouse and stimulate. It is a color that symbolizes warmth, active intelligence, self-confidence, gaiety, happiness, the joy of expression, and a cosmopolitan attitude. It is considered to be a color that inspires happiness, helps the person achieve self-confidence and realize intellectual abilities, and guards energy or incentive.

The color orange has a soothing and anti-spasmodic effect on the organism. From the physical point of view, orange has the ability to arouse gently, and to fortify the blood flow. It is linked to the spleen and pancreas, to the digestive system and kidneys, and is used for treating asthma, bronchitis, and a wide range of respiratory and pulmonary problems, stomach problems, pains in the joints, calcium problems, feminine problems (such as menstrual disorders, impaired fertility, sterility), muscle spasms, and so on. In addition, the color orange reinforces the metabolism.

From the emotional point of view, orange is used to help nervous or depressed states, since it arouses joy and gaiety (especially in situations of a complete lack of interest in life), dispels a lack of self-confidence, and helps when there is a lack of energy and enthusiasm. This color combines physical energy - like the color red - and intellectual qualities - like the color yellow. It especially fortifies the etheric body, and promotes health generally.

When orange appears in the aura in a balanced way, it attests to analytical thought, the ability to apply the intellect in a practical manner, inventiveness, an abundance of ideas, self-confidence, good intellectual abilities, high motivation, healing ability, self- and interpersonal communicative ability, and prosperity.

When orange appears in the aura in an unbalanced way, it attests to ignorance, aggressiveness, exaggerated ambitiousness, and competitive thinking.

Orange that tends to red may attest to passion, enjoyment, a need for action, idealism, pride, and, when it is less balanced, conceit.

Orange that tends to yellow may attest to a sharp intellect, a lot of self-confidence, diligence, persistence, and a good ability to use the intellect for practical and productive purposes.

Yellow

Yellow is the color of the third chakra, the solar plexus chakra. It stimulates the intellect, the memory, and a good mood, and symbolizes lightness and gaiety. It is a consoling and reviving color, and represents the intellect and the mind, organizational ability, discipline, personality, and ego. The color yellow stimulates the motor nerves, as well as muscle energy.

Since yellow is a combination of red and green waves, it is used to stimulate red energy, and for renewed production of green.

The action of the color yellow on the nervous system and the brain is extremely powerful. From the physical point of view, yellow is linked to the liver, the gallbladder, the stomach, the large and small intestines, the lungs, the prostate gland, the thyroid gland, and the bronchial tubes. The color yellow is used to treat psychological problems such as depression, melancholy, mental exhaustion, and the inability to concentrate. It is good for treating the digestive and nervous systems, stimulates hormone production, helps in situations where there is thyroid imbalance, stimulates the liver and the kidneys, has a beneficial effect on the intestines, the spleen, the stomach, and the bladder, and stimulates cleansing via the liver. In addition, yellow helps in problems of a weak memory, and in skin care and treatment. It fortifies the entire digestive system, stimulates the digestive juices and the flow of lymphatic fluids, strengthens the nervous system, and purifies the blood.

When the color yellow appears in the aura in a harmonious way, it attests to high intellectual capacities and a strong personality, a good organizational ability, discipline, knowledge, honesty, harmony, a well developed ability to learn, career-oriented, scientific, and business thinking, business acumen, and diplomacy.

When the color yellow appears in the aura in a disharmonious way, it attests to stubbornness, skepticism, a critical nature, exaggerated emotional control, cynicism, egoism, ignorance, laziness, intolerance, and sorrow.

Light yellow among the colors of the aura attests to openness, calmness, a strong personality, and freshness and clarity of thought.

Ocher (yellow that tends slightly to brown) among the colors of the aura may attest to stability, realism, frugality to the point of cheapness, tensions, authority, control, excessive discipline, and egoism.

Pink

Pink is one of the colors of the fourth chakra, the heart chakra. It is not one of the basic colors of the spectrum, but is a mixture of white (which is light that comprises physically all the colors of the spectrum) and red, but it has beneficial healing properties, and is used widely in color therapy.

Since pink is a combination of red, which is a stimulating color that symbolizes among other things passion and love, and white, which consists of all the colors and symbolizes the link to the divine and the cosmic, pink is a healing color that expresses cosmic love.

The color pink arouses affection, love, and the desire to give; it has a warming and enveloping effect on the mind, and helps to restore youth. It is customary to use it when treating conditions of a lack of self-love and a feeling of loneliness and being unloved.

It should not be used for treating nervous or quick-tempered people.

In the aura, the color pink attests to sensitivity, emotionalism, femininity, yearning, softness, and sometimes excessive sentimentality.

Green - the "natural" color

The color green, which is located between the two groups of colors - the warm colors and the cool colors - and is composed of a mixture of a warm color (yellow) and a cool color (blue), is considered to be a natural color.

The color green is considered to be the major color of the heart chakra (in addition to green, pink is also suitable for this chakra, but not for everyone). Green is considered to be the general color of health, and it is used for treating every health problem except cancer (since it encourages growth, and some people claim that it is liable to speed up the growth of existing malignant tumors). Green is a color that represents youth, freshness, growth, energy, balance, and hope. Green is the color of nitrogen, an element that constitutes the main component of the atmosphere and is essential for the formation of the bones, the muscles, and the other tissues. As a result, the color green is considered to be the optimal healing color. It stimulates growth and life, balances body and mind, soothes, strengthens, helps to overcome obstacles and begin on a new path, and symbolizes harmony and balance.

Green is made up of blue and yellow, and constitutes a balancing link between the warm colors, which stimulate and energize, and the cool colors, which soothe. It helps to balance the energies while balancing the state of disharmony, and helps to achieve a new, healthy structure. Since it symbolizes nature, and is one of the dominant colors in the plant world, it represents the harmonious cycle of nature, growth, and renewal.

The color green has a soothing effect on the sympathetic nervous system, alleviates pains, and soothes irritations. From the physical point of view, green is linked to the muscles, the bones, the bronchial tubes, and the lungs. It is good for treating problems concerning the heart and the circulatory system, it balances blood pressure and has an invigorating effect on the blood vessels. It stimulates the pituitary gland (the gland that is responsible for most of the hormonal activity in the body), and while doing that helps to balance the entire hormonal system. Because of its beneficial action on the hormonal system, its action is effective for soothing states of emotional imbalance. It encourages cell renewal and overall regeneration of the organism, fortifies the body in general, and after an illness or injury in particular, and helps to improve the absorption of oxygen in the body.

When the color green appears in the aura in a balanced way, it attests to the ability to accept things as they are, as well as to growth, hope, change and new creation, unity and balance of the body, mind, and spirit, good communication, linking up to nature and comprehending it, universal love, the ability to succeed in the care professions, the performing arts, gardening, and agriculture.

When the color green appears in the aura in an unbalanced way, it may indicate jealousy, envy, pessimism, lack of satisfaction, resistance to the natural course of life, artificiality, and over-sentimentality.

Yellow-green among the colors of the aura may attest to sympathy for other people, compassion, the ability to forgive, good communication, honesty, and the love of peace.

Dark green among the colors of the aura attests to an ability to express oneself and present oneself, an ability to adapt, and vitality; and on the other hand, materialism, and a capacity for fraud and cunning.

Turquoise is a color that is composed of blue and green, and may have a stronger tendency toward one of them. For this reason, it is considered to belong to both the throat chakra and the heart chakra. It is a soothing color, good for conditions of heat; it gives a feeling of protection, cools both physically and mentally, soothes nervousness, alleviates headaches, and helps in the treatment of burns. When it appears in the aura in a nice and balanced way, it may be indicative of healing powers.

Cool colors

All the cool colors - blue, indigo, and purple - have cooling and soothing properties. They are linked to the feminine energy - the yin - which symbolizes the negative pole, passivity, the element of water, and coolness.

Blue
The color blue is the color of the fifth chakra, the throat chakra. It symbolizes depth and inward withdrawal, coolness, truth, devotion, wisdom, rest, renewal, revival, purity, calmness, and sleep. Although it possesses the highest energy of all the colors of the spectrum, its effect on the entire organism is the most soothing of all. It has a beneficial effect on the nervous system, and helps to treat various problems at the root of which is impaired nervous functioning (it helps with problems that are considered organic). It helps to lower blood pressure and slow down the heart rate. It helps to strengthen and shrink tissues, and slows down the development of tumors. This color is also considered to be

the color of meditation, spiritual development, intuition, and the highest moral and spiritual measures.

The throat chakra, to which it is linked, is considered to be the first of the upper chakras, and the center of creative power, and the color blue helps to develop the powers of expression and creativity.

From the physical point of view, the color blue is linked to the organs of touch, nerve cells, the brain, the spinal cord, the skin, and the hair. In color therapy and healing, blue is also used for treating respiratory problems, throat infections, bruises and burns, and sensory and emotional disturbances, and for lowering fever and infections.

The color blue is considered to be the most important color in treating gynecological diseases, menstrual cramps, and menopausal problems.

From the emotional point of view, blue is used for various aspects of achieving calmness and release from tension, for problems of insomnia, and for developing spiritual understanding and faith. Exaggerated use of blue in treatment may cause certain people to feel fatigue, or even depressed. Sometimes this feeling is liable to be caused by being in a room that is painted blue or has blue furnishings, or by wearing blue clothing. On the other hand, a slightly "blue" atmosphere can help hot-tempered people, who find it hard to calm down, feel more tranquil and calm.

When the color blue appears in an aura in a balanced and harmonious way, it attests to love, wisdom, trust, truth, inner equilibrium, honesty, reliability, manners, rest, centering, confidence, tranquillity, patience, a forgiving nature, cooperation, sensitivity, seeing things correctly, belief, inner quiet and sometimes reticence, devotion, and awareness of the divine.

When the color blue appears in an aura in an unbalanced way, it may indicate exaggerated restraint, a lack of involvement, solitude and seclusion, fears and anxieties, depression, sadness, passivity, a lack of interest in what's going on, emotional coldness, and self-pity.

Light blue among the colors of the aura may attest to softness, attraction to religion or faith, dedication to ideas and beliefs, a certain conservatism, and sometimes voluntary solitude.

Indigo

Indigo is a mixture of dark blue and purple, and is considered to be the color of the sixth chakra, the third eye chakra. It symbolizes healing abilities, seriousness, politeness, morality, and purity of intentions. Indigo is the color that is in charge of the flow of the energy of the delicate body through the sixth chakra, which is the spiritual energy center.

On the physical, astral, and spiritual planes, indigo affects the visionary ability, as well as the senses of sight, hearing and smell. From the physical point of view, indigo is linked to the senses of hearing, sight, and smell, and the auditory, visual, and olfactory organs. It is used for treating problems of the nervous system, as well as problems connected to sight and hearing. Indigo helps with problems of fever that are connected to the lymph glands, and is very effective in purifying the circulatory system, in regulating metabolism and cell renewal in the body, and in treating cases of disturbances in the respiratory system.

A unique use of the color blue in color therapy is releasing the person from negative color loads that accumulated in the past. This treatment is performed by projecting the color indigo on the patient.

When indigo appears in the aura in a harmonious and balanced way, it attests to unity, inspiration, rest, balance, synthesis, inner tranquillity and peace, healing powers, and the ability to see auras and divine visions. (The color may occasionally appear in the auras of priests, psychologists, healers, and social workers.)

When indigo appears in the aura in a disharmonious way, it is liable to indicate pride, arrogance, exaggerated restraint, domination, and tyranny.

Purple

The color purple is attributed to the sixth chakra, the third eye chakra, as well as to the seventh chakra, the crown chakra. It represents intuition, art, creativity, extra-sensory abilities, belief, imagination, and non-corporeality. Purple is a color that grants inspiration, opens up spiritually, and reinforces meditative abilities.

The color purple has powerful healing properties, and also helps nervous problems and mental diseases, as well as problems in the person's mental body in cases in which it is necessary to stimulate or fortify the person's spiritual aspect.

From the physical point of view, the color purple is good for weight reduction, stimulating the spleen, increasing the production of leukocytes (white blood cells whose action is essential for the immune system), curbing diarrhea, and purifying the blood.

When the color purple appears in the aura in a harmonious and balanced way, it attests to powerful intuition, spirituality and spiritual abilities, extra-sensory abilities, the ability to receive spiritual messages and information, creativity, devotion, idealism, a calm attitude, a meditative and tranquil way of life, and the ability to change and develop.

When the color purple appears in the aura in a disharmonious way, it may attest to religious fanaticism, a lack of justice, obsessive behavior, intolerance of anything different, use of negative powers and black magic, belief in punishment and penalization, and impotence.

Lavender is lilac, a light and delicate purple. When it appears among the colors of the aura in a balanced and harmonious way, it may attest to mystical abilities, positive magical powers, and depth of thought.

When it appears in the aura in a disharmonious way, it is liable to indicate an obsessive nature, excessive fanaticism about ideas, and intolerance of anything different.

Magenta is a mixture of red and pink, and is considered to be one of the colors of the seventh chakra, the crown chakra. This color is thought to be a cosmic color, and attests to a cosmic healing ability.

In color therapy, magenta is used for treating problems concerning the brain, inspiration of happiness and vitality (in cases of a depressed mood), energizing, and treating infections and problems in the arteries and kidneys.

White

White is the color of the crown chakra, and of the high, pure energy. White light is created from the combination of all the colors of the spectrum, in the same way that white sunlight contains all the colors of the spectrum.

In color therapy, healing, and meditation, white is sometimes used to stimulate the transformation of the awareness, and for linking up to divine energy. When the color white appears in the aura in a harmonious and balanced way (this can be seen in many infants), it indicates a link to divinity, spirituality, and superior spiritual abilities, purity, filling up with light and energy, great and developed intelligence, and higher levels of awareness, enlightenment, and unity of all the colors.

When the color white appears in the aura in an unbalanced way, that is, in centers where it is not supposed to appear, such as in the lower chakras, or if it tends to look "dirty," or not harmonious, it is liable to attest to detachment from solid ground, daydreams, focal points of too much energy (a phenomenon that can indicate a painful place), a lack of centering, and the accumulation and absorption of energy in an unbalanced and uncontrolled way.

Complementary colors

Complementary colors are also called "contrasting colors," especially by painters. Each color of the spectrum has a complementary color. Many healers have discovered that an imbalance in the basic color is liable to create an imbalance in the complementary color. Therefore, many color therapists project the basic color for two-thirds of the therapy session, and the complementary color for the remaining third.

The complementary color of red is turquoise; the complementary color of green is magenta; the complementary color of blue is orange; the complementary color of purple is yellow; the complementary color of indigo is gold - and vice versa.

The use of complementary colors is important mainly when a dominant color such as blue or red is projected, transmitted, or conveyed to a person, since the stimulating action of the red is liable to be too extreme or too strong, causing certain people to become restless and nervous, while the calming and cooling action of the blue is liable to cause a feeling of fatigue and a downward moodswing.

Methods of treatment, identifying, finding, and radiating colors

The large body of knowledge concerning the action of colors that was presented in the previous chapters, and similarly, the additional knowledge about the color types that will be presented later on, is practical knowledge that can be used both for understanding, for increasing self-awareness, and for the comprehension of the people around us and close to us, as well as for treatment, change, growth, spiritual development, and broadening awareness,

There are numerous methods of treatment with color.

As we mentioned previously, color is used for treating both physical and emotional aspects, and, of course, for promoting spiritual development.

There are several accepted, useful, and easy methods of treatment with colors, but matching the personal color to the patient must be done in one of two ways that are commonly used and have proved themselves in practical application:

By reading the aura and gaining an accurate understanding of the nature of the color, the personal situation, or the patient's condition, and identifying the color that he lacks or needs.

By identifying the required color intuitively.

We discussed the significance of reading the aura in the first part of the book, and we will elaborate upon it in the third part.

Regarding the second way, remember that identifying the appropriate color intuitively requires spiritual openness and purity, and spiritual work has to be done before one can acquire the ability to receive messages intuitively.

Before we describe a number of methods for using colors and administering treatment with colors, we will suggest a few ways for identifying the required color intuitively. Of course, every healer, therapist, or layman can find the way that is suitable and right for him personally.

Finding the color that is necessary for you personally - a basic technique

This technique should not be applied after a heavy meal, in a state of extreme fatigue, or after an emotional crisis, unless you can detach yourself from your emotions and calm down.

Choose a quiet, calm, tranquil, and clean place in which to link up.

Sit, stand, or lie comfortably, with your body straight and comfortable. Close your eyes.

Breathe deeply, slowly, and comfortably several times.

Relax your entire body, starting with your toes, and progressing upward, releasing and relaxing every single organ.

In order to relax your body, you can breathe a conscious breath into every organ (simply inhale and imagine the air penetrating the organ; or think of the organ at the moment of inhalation).

In the same way, you can use the technique of contraction and relaxation - contract the organ hard, and then relax it entirely.

Continue breathing through your nose; be aware of your breathing.

When you have reached a meditative state, make the following request either aloud or clearly in your thoughts: "I would like to know what color I need now in order to balance and strengthen my aura."

The answer is likely to appear in many different ways. You may see a spot of color - or more than one - in front of your closed or open eyes, or a ray of light in the required color. You may see the name of the color (generally speaking, the letters of the name will be in that color), or you will suddenly have a clear insight, as though spoken by an inner voice, of the color/s you need.

I have been told by several people that at the moment of opening their eyes, a spot of the color appeared; or they noticed a certain object and its color just as they opened their eyes - and an inner insight made it clear to them that it was the color they needed.

Frequently, more than one color appears with this technique; and often, with great accuracy, the appropriate complementary colors also appear.

Receiving information via the "third eye"

This technique must be applied in the same way as the first basic technique, except that here, after relaxing the body and breathing consciously, the person must concentrate his awareness in the center between his eyebrows - the third eye - and repeat the declaration that he made in the basic technique. Alternatively, he can simply wait for the information.

It is preferable to breathe through the third eye until the appearance of the necessary color/s.

Matching the color to another person

This technique is also based on the basic technique, but in this case, you must attune yourself to the patient. This can be done by laying hands on the patient, sitting opposite him, and scrutinizing him before he closes his eyes and relaxes, or imagining him in your mind's eye, even if he is not present. You can also imagine his presence beside you. In this case, you must fill yourself with compassion, love, and caring, and be aware that you are requesting the color in order to help someone else. In the declaration, say: "I would like to know the color that is appropriate for ..... [say the patient's name lovingly] for his balance and health," or any similar declaration. You can also mention the disease or problem from which the person is suffering, and for which you are making the request. As in the previous techniques, the color will appear in front of your eyes, or you will feel intuitively what the appropriate color is. In any event, you must make it clear to yourself that you are requesting the appropriate color for someone else, and not for yourself. Don't get confused.

There are many other methods, such as using crystals, pendulums, or colored cards. These methods are simple, and the accessories serve merely as aids for focusing your awareness.

If for some reason you do not succeed in identifying the color intuitively, you should identify it with the help of the description of the significance of the colors in the previous and following chapters (in the analysis of the color types), and by means of question and analogy. In other words, question the person and find out what the most suitable color is for the given situation.

However, do not despair, and continue trying to find out what the color is intuitively, since ultimately it is likely to be the most correct and accurate one.

Projecting colors

When we begin describing the systems for healing and treatment with colors, we have to start with the method that is the most widespread among many healers, which is also the most effective method: projecting color.

Projecting a color is seeing the color in one's imagination, and projecting it to the patient (remember that the patient may also be the healer, or he may be a different person). It is a direct continuation of the technique of finding and identifying the color, and it is possible, for instance, to continue meditating and receiving the color and filling up with it immediately after the meditation for discovering the color intuitively.

A ray of colored light

When you have found out which color you need for balancing and strengthening the aura - yours or someone else's - imagine a ray of light of the same color coming down from above. If you do not perform this technique directly after asking the question concerning the color, you must relax your body and breath conscious breaths, until you feel tranquil and calm and ready to receive the color. The ray of light that comes down from above penetrates the crown of the head, fills the body and the organs with color, and, with each breath, continues filling the body, flowing down via the spinal column, and exiting the body through the soles of the feet into the depths of the earth.

The ray of light that is projected onto the patient (even without imagining the process of filling up) can be "held" for 15 to 20 minutes, or according to intuitive feeling. It is possible to project the complementary color of the main color onto the patient for about a third of the time, for the sake of maintaining the balance.

This method of treatment, simple as it seems, is effective and successful in most cases.

I recall an interesting case in which a young student of healing asked me to advise her how to help her boyfriend, who had suffered from premature ejaculation for many years (in fact, he did not know anything different...). Since the color blue is a calming and delaying color, I asked her to visualize in her mind's eye - while they were still dressed, before having sex - a ray of blue light directed at his genitals, soothing and balancing his sexual system, and at the same time inducing a state of overall positive calmness in him.

Projecting the color blue was extremely simple, and she

did it without her boyfriend even noticing. The results were astonishing. It was the first time in the young man's life that he did not suffer from that particular tiresome symptom. Of course, I was rewarded with an excited and grateful phone-call. In order to maintain the new situation and reinforce it, my student continued to project the blue light onto him every time they were about to have sex. With his success in "holding back" longer, his self-confidence increased, and his fears and anxieties about "failure" - premature ejaculation - which had done nothing but increase his problem, decreased until they disappeared altogether, while the couple's sex life blossomed, to their great delight.

Projecting via the hands

This technique is recommended for people who are already experienced in healing, Reiki, or other healing techniques. People who are unable to empty themselves of thoughts and feelings should not use it.

\# Sit opposite the person, or, if he is not present, imagine him in your mind's eye, or feel him sitting in front of you.

\# After emptying yourself of all thoughts and feelings, taking slow, deep conscious breaths, and feeling your body relaxed and free of all tension, and your head drained of all thought, think of the person, and see his name written in front of you in your mind's eye, or imagine it.

\# Feel how you become filled with energy.

\# Turn the palms of your hands toward the patient, and begin to project the color onto him, while you imagine in your mind's eye how the color releases the blockages in the person, and fills him, heals him, balances him, and makes him happy.

Before any attempt at healing, you should request help and assistance from the universal force, in order to ensure success, protection, and purity.

The ellipse of colored light

This technique is very similar to the previous one, except that here you see the patient (or yourself) surrounded by a large and beautiful ellipse of the required color. The ellipse protects and guards both you and the patient (if it is not a self-treatment) from undesirable influences, preserves his energies, strengthens him, and protects his health.

It is extremely important to know that in color therapy and healing, the color black is not used! It is not projected, and it is not sent. Sometimes, it is used in clothing in order to provide a feeling of protection, but it is not used in healing techniques.

As a result of its cleanliness and purity, the color white is very difficult to project, because it is not always possible to ensure that it will be projected clean and pure, therefore it too should not be projected (especially not at the beginning).

On the other hand, the color gold is good and suitable in every projection of color and color healing, because it is the universal and supreme healing color.

The color green, too, is suitable for treatment and projecting in every impaired physical state and for every health problem, except for tumors.

Methods of treatment for everyday use

1. Wearing clothes in the required color: As often as you can, you should wear clothes in the required color, or in two colors - the basic color and the complementary color. These could even be the two colors you like the least, but you need them more than anything.

If you discover that this is the situation, it would seem that you need to take a real serious look at your situation. In any event, don't fight the changes; wear the clothes in the colors you need, and try to remain aware while you wait for the changes and the feelings that arise in you as a result of wearing the clothes.

2. Eating foods in the required color: If the color you have selected is a color that is characteristic of various foods, fruits, or vegetables (of course, this doesn't mean foods that contain food coloring!), you should eat them. Examples include:

orange - pumpkin, yams, carrots

green - green vegetables of all kinds (no shortage of those!)

red - red peppers, tomatoes

purple - beets, grapes

yellow - grapefruit, lemons, bananas

and so on for each color for which foods can be prepared using natural ingredients.

Many healers, especially in Shaman and Chinese medicine, use this technique, which has proved to be effective.

3. The use of precious stones and crystals* in the required color: Precious stones and crystals have prodigious and extraordinary qualities that exert a significant action on the human organism in general, and on the electro-magnetic field in particular. Each stone has its unique properties, and its color is extremely significant.

When you know what color you need, you can find yourself a suitable crystal, even without any prior knowledge of its properties and qualities. All you have to do is to go to a New Age store and look at stones in the color you need. Concentrate and direct yourself at your purpose - finding a stone that will help you complete whatever is lacking in your aura, in order to strengthen it, and for your general balance. Choose the stone that appeals to you the most and purchase it. This is the simplest and most effective way, since stones have the ability to join up with you, and we can know intuitively, without conscious thought, which stone is appropriate for us.

After you have selected your stone, make inquiries about it; there is every chance that you will be surprised to discover how well it suits you.

After purchasing the stone, find out from the salesperson whether it is possible to purify it in salt water, and if it is permitted to used it as a potion. Do not do these things without checking first, because there are stones that are destroyed as a result of contact with salt, and there are stones that contain poisonous minerals and *must not* be used as potions.

* *The concepts "stone," "precious stone," and "crystals" - in holistic arts indicate stones that originate in the earth, and are used for purposes of awareness. Pearls, mother-of-pearl, fossilized wood and so on (that do not originate in the earth) are also called by these names.*

After purchasing the stone, place it in water mixed with sea salt for three hours. Then place it on the windowsill for 24 hours.

Do not use a stone without purifying it! One of the properties of stones is the absorption of energy, and you do not want to take in the energies of all the people that excavated it, handled it, and traded it. After purifying it, you can use the stone in any way you want: You can hold it in your hand, meditate with it, place it on any organ on which you feel the need to put it, carry it in your pocket, wear it, and if it a stone from which a potion may be prepared (and it is of an appropriate size), it can also be sucked like a sweet.

Preparing a potion from the stone is very simple and effective. Place the stone in a transparent glass, and fill the glass with mineral water. After the preparation, place the glass on the windowsill for three hours, so that it can absorb the sun's rays, thus completing the full extraction of the energetic color. Afterwards, remove the stone and drink the water.

Let us emphasize once more how important it is to ensure that it is permissible for the stone to be used for preparing a potion.

In any event, after using the stone, it must be purified under cold running water for about five minutes, since it probably absorbed your non-positive energies, as well as giving you its energies, so it needs to be strengthened and refreshed. Crystals must be treated with respect and gratitude, in the same way as you would relate to your physician, holistic healer, or teacher.

Of course, there are many different and creative ways to fill your life with the color you need for strengthening your aura. In general, try to "envelop" yourself in objects, items of clothing, and accessories of the required color, hang fabrics of the suitable color on the walls, and if you feel a significant and strong lack of the color, you can even paint the room in which you spend most of your waking hours in that color. Gradually, you will begin to feel the change and the influence of the color on your physical and mental state.

When you feel a decline in your mood or in your general feeling, take a ribbon or a piece of paper of your required color, and stare at it for a few minutes.

An additional method, which is recommended for a quick and effective treatment, is to sit or lie opposite a light-bulb of your required color, or wrapped in cellophane paper of that color, for about 10-15 minutes, or according to how you feel (if you are in tune with your feelings, you will know precisely when you are sufficiently "full" of your color). It is always a good idea to combine two complementary colors, projecting the basic color for about three quarters of the treatment time, and the complementary color for the remaining quarter, so as to maintain balance, and prevent a situation in which too much color is projected - either generally or at that specific time.

After you learn the color types, whose characteristics will be described in the next section, you will be able to use the knowledge you have obtained to raise your awareness, and to vary your colors, thus promoting your physical, mental, and spiritual development. As we mentioned, you can also use this knowledge to identify and match up the colors you or other people need.

Color Types

As we mentioned previously, while our electro-magnetic field contains all the colors of the spectrum, it may be dominated by a particular color.

This color - the dominant color - expresses various personal, physical, mental, and spiritual traits, and determines the person's color type.

The person's color type - that is, the most dominant color in his aura over a long period of time - governs his behavior, social skills, aspirations, aims, passions, mode of action - in fact, his entire personality, "who he is." When a person is aware of his color type, he can better understand his personality, passions, and motives, as well as his inner conflicts and the factors that hold him back or impede his progress.

Many people experience great relief when they understand that certain behavior patterns or conflicts are the expression of their color type, and that they have the ability to control the situation and even change it to suit themselves. As a result of such insights, the person can also live his life by associating with any color he wants, because of his aspiration to be a multifaceted person, and reach a state in which all the colors in his aura glow at balanced frequencies, causing his personality to resonate in all the colors of the rainbow.

If you are not blessed with the ability to see your aura, and you do not know what the dominant color in your aura is, you should read the characteristics of each color type in order to find the one to which you belong. In general, the relevant color type jumps out at you, clear and obvious. If you are vacillating between several types, read the material again, and check which of the basic points suit you the most.

There are a dozen basic color types:

**DARK RED * RED * YELLOW BROWN * YELLOW
ORANGE * GREEN * DARK GREEN * BLUE *
INDIGO * PURPLE * LAVENDER * WHITE ***

The dark red personality type - the worker

People of the dark red type are earthy, realistic, and practical, and have a great deal of physical strength. They link up well to the physical stratum of reality, and live their lives intensively and powerfully. They relate easily to the material, physical world, and love to discover and try out the many possibilities that it offers them from the physical and material points of view. It is not easy to convince a dark red type of the existence of other strata of being and reality, because this type only believes what he can see, touch, taste, smell, and hear.

From the physical point of view, people of this type are generally well-built, with a strong, stable body that they love to activate and move. Physical activity is not a pastime for them, but rather a way of life. People of this type feel unbalanced when they are prevented from activating and moving their bodies and giving free rein to their physical strength, because they need opportunities to express this strength in order to feel balanced and centered. They enjoy hard physical labor and are accustomed to it; they feel "at home" in a job that permits them to use their strength. They also love sports of all kinds. The earth energy that flows in these types must be channeled by means of enormous and powerful activation of their body. "Heavy" sports such as boxing and body-building, and every other kind of powerful, impulsive physical activity, constitute excellent ways for expressing the strong earth energy that characterizes them.

Similar to the base chakra, whose color is red, people of the dark red type focus on survival and safeguarding what exists. In a harmonious state, people of this type have qualities of great physical power, the ability to preserve the present, reliability, stability, and honesty; they are faithful workers who are always prepared to do hard, strenuous work.

When people of this type are balanced, they are courageous, full of *joie de vivre*, and eager to cope with challenges. From the mental point of view, they are down-to-earth, think in a practical manner, and tend to be conservative. They eschew activities that demand abstract or complex thought, or require that they believe in things that cannot be perceived via their five senses. When abstract, philosophical ideas, or ideas that are not firmly anchored in their concept of reality are propounded, they display intolerance, and feel emotional and even physical unease. Most of their power lies in their understanding of physical and material reality, and in this area, they can notch up many achievements, and display serious and sincere interest.

Since they are not interested in hearing new ideas or different philosophies, these types are liable to follow the world view that they acquired in their childhood blindly, slavishly, and unquestioningly. Living and acting in accordance with the accepted laws of society provides dark red types with a feeling of security; they need these laws in order to feel that they are in fact operating in the correct way and are doing "what has to be done."

People of this type love to center their strength and express it in hard work that yields immediate results. It is very important for them to receive clear and visible results. For this reason, a situation occasionally arises in which they exhaust themselves with overwork and too much activity in order to obtain the results right away, and this is liable to cause them frequent states of pressure and tension. They do not find it easy to throw in the towel, relax, and calm down, even when the situation requires it. Overwork and hyperactivity are par for the course in the lives of people of this type (especially when they are not balanced). They are constantly busy and active, always in a hurry, and sometimes work at several jobs or occupations simultaneously; in the "best" case, they move on to another task as soon as they finish the previous one.

Their deepest fears are of poverty and death. Their economic situation and financial security for them and their families constitute their top priorities. These topics bother them and sometimes cause them to get caught up in the pursuit of financial security - a result of the feeling that their lives and survival depend on it.

Despite the forcefulness that people of this type project - both from the physical and the behavioral points of view - they are basically warm and sensitive people.

Unfortunately, however, they sometimes tend to conceal their feelings, so that other traits that characterize them, such as a hot temper and outbursts of anger, erupt very frequently in their lives. Their ability to give vent to their feelings very naturally is sometimes liable to manifest itself as a lack of consideration, and acting delicately is far beyond their capabilities. The moment they feel the need to express their "external" feelings, their emotions burst out in a powerful and impulsive manner that is difficult to curb. Frequently, people of this type feel the urge to express their feelings physically, and this is liable to lead to physical conflict.

On the other hand, these people are liable to internalize their inner feelings, and sometimes not even be aware of them! It is difficult for them to speak about their inner feelings, to share them, and to open up.

Health, growth, and development

As we mentioned previously, people of the dark red type are blessed with an enormous abundance of emotional and physical energy, and when they do not find positive outlets for it, they are liable to get into one of two situations: outbursts of fury and violence, or depression and a lack of will to live. For some reason, they are inclined to view the expression of emotions as "weak," "childish," "not masculine," and so on, and for that reason, they frequently reject their emotions. Hiding and repressing their emotions makes them appear brutal, insensitive, noisy, and sometimes even dangerous.

One of the most important lessons that people of this type must learn is to express their emotions in positive ways, to release their energies via athletic or creative outlets, and to accept their emotions as natural and normal, as things that can be discussed and expressed, with no fear of hurt or rejection.

They are the only ones who can create a channel of positive and harmonious expression both for venting their energies and for inducing a state of calm, release, and relaxation for themselves. It is very difficult for them to calm down, empty their heads of all thoughts, and stop running from one activity to the next, but this calmness is vital to them. If they don't learn to calm down, they are soon liable to feel listless, nervous, or depressed. For this reason, they must find some kind of athletic activity, creative outlet, dynamic way of relaxing, or other way of calming down and releasing energy, in conjunction with accepting and understanding their emotions and learning to express them without fear.

One of the factors that most inhibits people of this type is the fear of death, loneliness, and poverty. The more this type of person's way of thinking is negative and pessimistic, the more these fears, even if they are unconscious, tend to affect their lives, and take on a realistic shape. To tell the truth, it is not easy to convince these people of the importance of positive declarations (see the chapter about the mental body), but it is exactly the use of this kind of declaration - "I love and esteem myself," "I feel secure and protected," "I express my feelings easily and lovingly," "My feelings are natural and acceptable" - that will bring these people ineffable calmness, tranquillity and happiness. As a rule, trusting in life, in God, in human beings, and in the universe, as well as an attitude that is positive and full of *joie de vivre* are the ways that will lead people of this type to fully realize their potential, and to enjoy a satisfying, happy life.

Accepting their feelings as natural and acceptable will enable them to express them and share them with the people close to them, and will, at the same time, help them to accept other people's feelings. This is vitally important for maintaining a harmonious, caring, and sensitive relationship. Living in fear and the survival instinct are the things that cause people of this type to get caught in a situation of emotional and spiritual stagnation, a situation that is focused on the fears of the first chakra. The moment they understand that they are the ones who are responsible for guiding their lives, like all human beings, and that they live in a universe in which the freedom of choice is the innate right of every person, people of this type will experience marvelous mental and spiritual growth and openness. Together with their enormous strength, power and energy, they will become useful, essential, loved and loving members of the human fabric of the universe. Despite the fact that this point of view seems so alien to them, and the concept "spiritual development" does not seem to apply to them, this is not the case! All they have to do is direct the focus of their energies away from survival, struggle, and fear, to channels that are characterized by creativity and initiative. When they understand that life is more than eating, working, sleeping, and having sex, that it consists of many different and fascinating strata, which are special and full of emotion, they can direct their energies to development, growth, and mental balance, which will cause them to reach above themselves and experience life to the full.

Because they are so physical and full of strength, they may begin these processes with their body - by means of athletic activities that include a step into the mind and spirit. In fact, there are many people of this type who, by learning Oriental martial arts that lead them to undergo far-reaching mental and spiritual growth.

Since people of this type are inclined to be so intense, and invest so much strength and power in everything they do - occasionally to the point of exhaustion - they should focus on healthy and correct nutrition combined with regular physical activity. Although many of them are partial to beef, beer, and heavy, fatty foods, lighter, fat-free vegetarian dishes are more likely to begin to lead to that wonderful mental change that they are yearning for deep in their hearts. The food we eat has an enormous effect on the equilibrium not only of our bodies, but also of our minds, and people of this type must take care to eat correctly.

The red personality type - the winner

You often come across people of this type in the administrative offices of large companies. Because they are powerful, energetic, gifted with extraordinary will power, great leadership ability, and a tremendous desire to succeed, people of this type are likely to occupy senior positions in the business world. Although people of the red type tend to live their lives in the here and now, enjoying everything the material world has to offer to the full, they are practical and realistic, and admire successful, competitive, and powerful people. Their motto in life is success, and they do everything to achieve it. They also have the qualities for doing so - single-mindedness, practicality, determination, perseverance, and a strong urge to create and make their lives into something very significant and tangible.

Just like the element of fire, which represents them, they are full of passion and excitement, and aspire to broaden the arena of their physical control. They do this very courageously and self-confidently. A life devoid of enthusiasm is liable to quench the fire that burns in them. The more their lives are filled with enthusiasm, passion, and excitement, the better and more vital they will feel. Life that lacks meaning - and for them, meaning is success - is not life. They are motivated by an uncontrollable urge to achieve clear and tangible results, to succeed and win, and because of their fierce will power and almost limitless physical energy that enables them to be exceptionally active, they frequently succeed in accomplishing their objectives.

The practical expression of their forceful energy contributes to their equilibrium and good feeling. A competitive and successful work environment, which is liable to stress other types out, causes people of the red type to feel that they are in the correct place - a place that permits them to face fascinating and stimulating challenges, and to prove to everyone - especially to themselves - that they can be successful and victorious in anything they choose to do.

People of the red type need interest, action, and new experiences in their lives. Routine that lacks "fire" and new, fascinating facts to satisfy their boundless curiosity about a vast range of topics makes them very frustrated. They like instant gratification, and know how to get it. Tolerance is not their strong suit.

They work toward accomplishing their goals with determination and assertiveness, and thanks to their prodigious will power - together with their strong physical and emotional energies - they are usually hugely successful in today's competitive and materialistic society. Other people may feel that these properties, as well as the strength that these people embody, are too intense, and sometimes even stressful, because their strength is manifested both on the physical and on the emotional planes.

Health, growth, and development

People of the red type have strong, active physical and emotion energy. Unlike most of the other color types, they do not suffer from a lack of energy. On the contrary: They have to learn to find positive and creative outlets into which to channel their energy. People of this type have a hard time winding down; in fact, it is well-nigh impossible to get them to wind down, relax, and rest. For this reason, they should find an activity that permits them to wind down. Activities such as jogging, swimming, dancing, and other types of physical exercise can help them relax and clear their heads, without making them feel frustrated that they "are sitting around doing nothing."

People of the red type feel that in order to live harmonious and satisfying lives, they need to realize all of their tremendous potential. Sometimes, after achieving a particular objective that they worked toward with every fiber of their being, they feel empty, and immediately look for the next objective to be conquered, the next challenge to be met. But it is extremely important for them to direct their plentiful energies at the right targets; no less important is for them to understand that winning is not everything in life, and winning at any cost is sometimes liable to take its toll in victims and hurting others.

People of this type must learn to release their tremendous energies without hurting others. Not infrequently, in moments of frustration and anger, the enormous fire that symbolizes this type is liable to burst forth and burn anyone in its path. It is vital for these people to display understanding and sensitivity toward the various needs and ways of other people. Just as importantly, they must be sufficiently sensitive to feel and accept their own feelings. If they learn to accept other people's feelings, to behave more gently with others, and to give free rein to their feelings - by sharing them more openly, instead of repressing them until there is an explosion - they will feel more love and acceptance in their lives, and will enjoy a more harmonious, tranquil, and loving environment.

They must learn to express their feelings in a creative way by means of calming physical activity, instead of repressing and concealing them below the surface. Furthermore, they must learn to channel their powerful energy and tremendous excitement into positive paths such as athletic activities, working out, physical work, or creativity. Creative ways of expressing their need for action fill them with energy and recharge their large energy reserves.

The yellow-brown personality type - the scientist

People of the yellow-brown type are stable, responsible, and exude a feeling of confidence into their surroundings. They are rational, analytical, creative, and consistent in their thinking. Their motivation in life is to understand life - in an analytical and intellectual way - and to communicate with the rest of the human race.

As we said before, their strongest qualities are their clear thinking and their analytical and logical abilities; they like to view life as a computer - you program the computer, input the data, and receive output. It is important to them to construct a stable foundation for their activities, because it gives them confidence. They examine every step they take carefully, moving on to the next stage only after thoroughly examining the results of the previous stage and whatever is involved in the next one - until they accomplish their final objective. Everything they do is logical and systematic, and they are constantly planning and meticulously examining the steps that are required for accomplishing their aim.

People of this type use their intellect all the time - they live by it, generally speaking. One could say that they use their bodies and emotions less than people of the other color types, and that most of their focus is on the intellectual aspect of life. They do not consider physical activity particularly important, and will only move their bodies if they think that there is a clear reason and advantage in doing so.

In their communication with other people, and their way of expressing themselves, people of this type are slow and considered. They describe every situation in minute detail, with a great deal of deliberation. They prefer to talk about their thoughts and ideas, as well as the projects they are involved in. They are very cautious when expressing their deep feelings and emotions, and will share these with other people only when they are absolutely convinced that the information will not be used against them, or hurt them in any way.

People of this type like to work and play around with electronic instruments, cars, mechanical equipment, and so on. They like to know all the little details, and when they are involved in a particular occupation or pastime, they get down to basics, and usually become experts on the subject. As a general rule, they are experts in their field. People of this type are among the developers of computers, electronics, and many technological instruments; this is because of the enormous amount of patience that characterizes them, their focus on detail, their determination, and their relentless pursuit of their goal.

These people have a clear perception and view of their lives. They do not like things that seem abnormal, out of the ordinary, or exceptional. Because of their love of security, they are inclined to stick to old patterns, and to tried and tested ways of thinking. They like a fixed daily routine and regular habits, and stick to them. For this reason, they sometimes find it difficult to accept new ideas, new patterns, and encounters with the unexpected. However, their stable, secure, and comfortable way of life is envied by many people in our society, especially by people in the business world.

People of this type are liable to have a problem accepting their emotions. They tend to examine feelings analytically, as if they were their own psychologists or analysts, instead of feeling them. Occasionally they are afraid of their own emotions, since these emotions prove that not everything in the world can be defined rationally and logically. The fear and insecurity run so deep that people of this type sometimes use sure, tried, tested, and old-fashioned modes of action to solve most of their problems! They feel safe with the same clear and stable modes of action and conduct that their parents, friends, and acquaintances routinely use, because that fact reassures them that these modes are innocuous.

Because they occasionally find it difficult to cope with their emotions, people of this type are liable to repress them and convince themselves that the emotions don't exist at all. They tend to make their emotions "disappear" in order not to have to deal with them. When they cannot accept and express their emotions, they are liable to become even more detached, cold, and unfeeling toward other people. When they repress their emotions, and internalize feelings such as sadness, anger, or frustration, they remain in a painful state of depression, hopelessness, and helplessness.

Health, growth, and development

For a person of this type, the first step toward equilibrium and harmony is getting in touch with his emotions. He has to learn to open up emotionally, and to begin to feel his and other people's emotions. This step demands a lot of courage from people of the yellow-brown type, but when they achieve this emotional openness and link-up, they are not only able to use their brains, but also to take advantage of the enormous strength that resides in their emotions. Emotional openness leads this type of person to acknowledge that intuition is an extremely important and vital aspect of life. The link-up to their intuition means living life with an open mind, and acknowledging new and unusual paths and ideas. Furthermore, it requires the willingness to reveal their full potential. They have to understand that skepticism results from a fear of change and a lack of security, and they have to learn to open themselves up to change and to new fields without always seeking information, facts, and tangible proof.

They must remain flexible, and be prepared to take risks. When these types maintain open horizons and emotional openness, they may enjoy tremendous success, and hold extremely important positions in society. They must remember that almost all the inventions and innovations were created and developed by people with an open mind and intuitive abilities.

If people of this type understand that reason is just a part of their personalities, they will rise above their fear of a lack of security. They must understand that their brains do not control them, but rather that they control their brains. With the help of this insight, they will calm down from this relentless rational process, and will discover their personalities and personal identities in a more profound manner.

People of this type must understand that making physical, mental, and emotional changes does not mean that things have gotten out of control. The world is in a state of constant change; change is one of the stages of growth, and it means taking true responsibility for life. By making significant but slow changes in life, people of this type increase their strength and power. When they liberate themselves from fear, and link up to their inner guide - their intuition and their deep inner emotions - they increase their vital energy and become the strong, spiritual creatures that they really are.

The understanding of life energy and of the different bodies that comprise the human being - the physical, etheric, emotional, mental, intuitive and spiritual bodies (see the chapter on the energetic bodies) - is very important to people of this type, and they must understand that all the bodies are equally important.

Because of their fear of taking risks, a large part of the inner strength of people of this type is not expressed. When they free themselves of the fear of a lack of stability, a lack of security, and a loss of control, and open up rationally and emotionally, they discover within themselves tremendous new inner powers that are liberated by the expression of their emotions and feelings in a clear and open way.

Excellent ways of opening and developing the spiritual and emotional energies of these types include creativity, dancing, singing, drawing, and all the other active, extrovert, and creative activities. Through calm, quiet meditation, and meditation with crystals, they will probably arrive at a passage leading to the strata of "regular" thought, to unlimited cosmic abilities, and openness to cosmic energy.

The yellow personality type - the entertainer

People of this type are the happiest, the most radiant, and the most childlike (in the positive sense of the word) of all the color types of the spectrum.

They are blessed with a flexible, flowing, light, and - similar to the sun - illuminating and warm personality. They have a marvelous sense of humor, love fun and laughter, and enjoy life in every possible way. They live their lives in a spontaneous way, and believe that life and work should always cause pleasure and happiness. These types will always remind the people around them "not to forget to enjoy life," and to see the half-full glass.

The factors that motivate people of the yellow type are enjoyment, creativity, entertainment, and fun. In their eyes, a good life is a life full of happiness and enjoyment. For them, a successful person is one who does what he likes to do, and devotes a lot of time to his pleasures. Their definition of success is: "Be creative, enjoy whatever you do, and achieve your aims while enjoying every step toward them."

People of this type are very energetic, and it is difficult for them to sit still for any length of time. When they are forced to do so, they fidget endlessly with their hands and with various objects, and make funny movements with their bodies. When they are nervous, frustrated, or irritated, they have to express their feelings immediately in order to liberate the strong current of energy that is flowing through them.

The bodies of people of this type are exceptionally sensitive. They can easily sense the feelings of those around them, and the energies in the room, and they are very open to everything that happens. Seeing that their senses are very open, they sometimes find that they are physically exhausted, without understanding why. The amount of information and activity that they "absorb," even subconsciously, is liable to exhaust their sensitive bodies.

Because they unconsciously use an extremely strong and clear body language, it is very easy to discern when they are happy, sad, or uncomfortable.

Their bodies constitute a measure of truth for their feelings, and they are blessed with an exceptional ability to sense and touch - which explains whey they frequently choose to work in the massage and healing professions. These professions are satisfying to them because of their love of helping people as well as being in the company of people. *Joie de vivre*, together with their healing abilities, makes them into excellent practitioners.

Health, growth, and development

The sensitive body of the yellow type of person resembles an energetic antenna, which ceaselessly picks up energetic messages from people around him, and from his surroundings. His body is extremely sensitive, and reacts very powerfully to external influences. More than people of any other color type, the yellow type has to worry about his body, give it the attention it deserves, and recognize its power in its many reactions, in order to use the information that it transmits to him as a means of protecting his health. If he does not look after his energy, from all points of view, his body is liable to be overly influenced by the external surroundings, and to show serious signs of imbalance.

People of this type are living proof of the link between the mind and the body. A lack of mental balance is expressed in a blatant way in the health of their bodies, so they have to learn to listen to their bodies and be aware of their mental state, their feelings, and their thoughts, all of which affect their overall health.

People of this type must learn that problems do not disappear if you ignore them or run away from them. They have to learn to cope with their problems by means of their innate happiness and their easy-going and flexible attitude to life, and understand that emotional obligation, as much as it may seem "threatening" to them or to their freedom and independence, will bring them joy and satisfaction, and will help their spiritual development. A profound relationship with their partners will lead them to very high levels of intimacy and self-awareness.

In order to feel harmonious and balanced, people of this type must expend their energy in creative activities, and express themselves through creation and joy. They have to find ways to express themselves both physically and creatively. They can balance their characteristic tendency to become addicted to certain things with "positive" addictions, such as athletic activities, meditation, prayer, healthy and enjoyable sex, movement, and trips. It is a good idea for them to become accustomed to enjoyable activities such as tennis, bicycle riding, jogging, and other physical activities that activate the muscles on a daily basis, in order to safeguard their health and channel their energy in a correct and beneficial way.

Dynamic meditations such as Tai Chi and the other activities that focus on the link between mind and body and bring about a link-up with the universal energy, are very beneficial for people of the yellow type. Moreover, they must recognize their healthy need for enjoyable and satisfying sexual intercourse in order to be joined to their energy bank and to stimulate their *joie de vivre*.

The orange personality type - the adventurer

You can meet many people of this type on the pages of history books - explorers, conquerors, inventors, and discoverers - especially in fields in which the person had to face dangers, overcome tremendous obstacles, and explore the unknown. People of this type are the most adventurous of all the color types. They are extremely creative, with a fierce urge to create, and they are independent and individualistic. They need excitement and enthusiasm in their daily lives, and combine intellectual qualities and physical abilities.

People of this type love to imagine and plan strategies for conquering their new target, or for devising a new adventure, and realizing these plans and strategies. In contrast to the lavender types, for example, these types love to be involved in the application of their ideas, and to help in the process of turning an idea into a reality. They feel the need to accompany the process from beginning to end, and it is difficult for them to stand to one side and see other people applying their ideas, or doing things for them. They are always busy with planning, designing, organizing, and constructing their projects on the conceptual and physical levels.

The principal motive in the life of people of the orange type is deriving pleasure and satisfaction from creating their own reality, from their adventures, and from life according to their ideas and perceptions. Furthermore, they derive pleasure and satisfaction from the process in which their ideas are realized. In contrast to people of other color types who work a great deal with their heads and with the conceptual aspect, these people are unable to sit and sketch ideas for other people to execute. They must be involved in the practical side of the realization of their ideas.

Because of this link between idea and execution, and because of the tremendous need of people of this type to prove to themselves and to others that they can cope with any challenge they face, they succeed in realizing their creative projects in an extraordinary way. All the necessary components for success and for turning an idea into a material and tangible reality are found in their characters. To conquer, to overcome every obstacle, to attain the impossible, to face new challenges that are placed before them by physical reality or by their own brains - all these are what motivate people of this type. It is extremely important for them to prove to themselves, and to others, that they are in control of their lives and reality, and they that achieve and create their own success.

Control - over their reality, thoughts and emotions - is an essential need of people of this type. To release, to relax, and to wind down are perceived by them as a loss of control - and for this reason, it is not easy for them to free their minds and bodies, or to sit quietly and do nothing. They are active all the time, intellectually or physically, and need to feel that they are constantly creating in thought, plan, or action. They are tightly linked to physical reality, and they experience life as if it were full of adventures, constant interest, and action.

People of this type channel their energies into the enjoyment of the physical world and its adventures. They need thrills, excitement, and constant challenges, and often relish the feeling of danger and "walking on the edge." Physical challenges such as mountain-climbing, swimming lakes, and many other challenges that most people would shy away from - and better still, challenges that no one else has yet managed to overcome - fascinate and excite people of this type in the extreme. They are liable to get into dangerous situations - physical or emotional - just so that they can feel that they are "more alive," or test their limits. The rush of adrenaline in the face of danger, from the new discovery or as a result of the unknown, is one of the favorite sensations of people of this type.

Nowadays, when man feels that he has already "taken control" of nature, when most of the world has already been "discovered" and surveyed, when the conquest of territories and countries is not as common as it was in the past, the characteristics of this type are not required for these purposes. Further back in history, these characteristics would place people of the orange type at the head of states and armies.

Moreover, the need for physical survival, which afforded these people countless opportunities to use their energy in everyday life - as hunters and warriors - has been translated nowadays into the need to "survive" economically, and to "fight" on the career, financial, and creative levels. For this reason, people of this type actively seek out opportunities that will enable them to channel their adventurous energy into action, either by means of challenging athletic activity, or by initiating daring projects.

Having said that, many people of this type prefer to channel their blazing adventurous energy into the field of mental creativity rather than into physical challenges. The possibility of adventure and creativity in the fields of enterprise and projects is more significant nowadays. People of this type prefer to expend their physical and intellectual energy in the creation and physical application of daring, innovative, exciting, challenging projects. They are very courageous, and love to establish new companies by themselves, do business and sell products, plan strategies, and carry out enterprises and deals.

They prefer to be the ones at the top, and execute their ideas, but they are not afraid of working on the finer details. It is important to them to be involved in the execution of their projects, and to apply things physically.

Health, growth, and development
In order to develop - to grow physically, mentally, and spiritually - and reach higher personal awareness, people of this type have to learn to see the "inner side" of their lives, and not just the "outer side," which they tend to see much more easily. People of this type must understand that equilibrium means the balance of the body, mind, and spirit, and not just one of those aspects. They must understand that in the world we live in, every action is significant, and egocentricity, hurting people, and trampling others underfoot affect the entire universe, and may even have a boomerang effect on the culprit. While they are busy looking for new challenges, people of this type sometimes forget the bigger challenge that faces human beings: the challenge of self-discovery, an adventurous journey that is no less challenging than white-water rafting, and requires the same courage as a bungy jump does, and the same determination as the conquest of a high mountain does.

Sometimes, in moments of deeper awareness, people of this type realize that they have hurt people more than once, or have displayed brusqueness or insensitivity toward others. Occasionally - and it is imperative that they know this - they adopt a defeatist attitude of "that's how I am, that's my character; I can't do anything about it." But they should know that the moment they delve more deeply into themselves, into the turbulent river of their mind, sit quietly in its depths, and feel the emotional storms that are raging overhead, they will receive exactly the information they need in order to understand how to change their personalities in a flowing and natural way, and will understand intuitively how to behave and how not to behave, and how to maintain beneficial relationships and contacts that do not hurt anyone else with themselves and with others.

When people of this type tune into their feelings, and learn to understand and know themselves, they will be able to understand and validate the feelings of people around them as well. Support of those around them, caring, openness, and sensitivity toward the rest of mankind will turn people of this type into essential and useful members of society - people who have the ability to change society and benefit humanity.

When people of this type learn to look at their inner side, to accept and understand feelings and sensitivities, a natural need will arise in them to channel their powerful energies into benefiting others, while the need, which is harmful at times, to create dangerous situations or to take risks in order to feel more "alive," will be replaced by the ability to use their tremendous strength to overcome every obstacle, in order to increase their own and the rest of humanity's knowledge, success, and satisfaction. People of this type are likely to give wonderful gifts to mankind, such as taking astounding photographs of the ocean floor, saving lives, and participating in rescue and aid delegations throughout the world. Their forceful adventurous energies are essential for the whole of mankind in many different fields.

Because of their extremely active nature, both physical

and mental, people of this type must be well aware of their emotional and physical condition, and see that they receive correct, healthy, and sufficient nutrition, as well as rest and relaxation. The creation of an environment that affords people of this type the freedom of creation and expression, together with making social and family contacts, is extremely important and significant for maintaining their harmonious and balanced state.

The green personality type - the teacher

The color green, which is situated in the center of the spectrum, between the warm and the cool colors, symbolizes equilibrium and harmony. This is how people of this type are, too - balanced, harmonious, and tranquil. They like to be in green surroundings, and are closely connected to nature; this closeness is very important to them. They prefer to live in the countryside, in villages, near bodies of water such as the sea, a river, or a lake, or near a park or a forest. People of this type are extrovert, open, friendly, and generous, and communicate with other people easily and warmly. In the same way that the color of the heart chakra is green, so people of this type experience the world through their hearts. Their definition of success is the ability to achieve proper equilibrium in life, as well as proximity to friends and to nature. Equilibrium and harmony are the major motivating factors in their lives. Inner happiness, satisfaction, and tranquillity are very important to them, and they do not need much, in material terms, to achieve them.

Although these people, like everyone, enjoy comfort and

luxury, they are neither competitive nor overly ambitious, and they do not chase after flashy clothes or fancy cars. They are aware of the fact that if they set themselves goals that are too high, they will have to make too much of an effort and experience too many difficulties to accomplish them. Because of their ability to understand the cycle and laws of nature, they consider human life to be the most wonderful gift of all.

People of this type are very talkative. They are very direct, say exactly what they are thinking, and can talk about any subject for hours, sometimes without saying too much... However, long conversations and heart-to-heart talks have a therapeutic effect on them; they need to talk about themselves, their feelings, and their problems in order to understand them in depth and to feel better. In the same way, they cannot restrain themselves when they are frustrated or feeling bad, and say exactly what they are feeling and thinking, since they cannot contain their emotions and thoughts without expressing them verbally. People of this type express emotion clearly and naturally. Anger, sadness, joy - all of these are expressed in their pure and clear form. Their emotional energies must be expressed, and they cannot repress them. They do not think about emotions, but rather express them.

Similar to the function of the heart chakra, people of this type also show that the true expression of feelings, without repressing them, hiding them, or resorting to manipulations, will probably lead to emotional equilibrium and harmony, which is their main aspiration. This emotional openness frequently permits them to live harmonious and natural lives, with excellent communication between them and their surroundings.

People of the green type have high and clear expectations from life. This is manifested mainly in their relationships with people and in their financial situation. They are not especially ambitious, and are not fond of hard work, but expect life to flow according to the way they want. They prefer natural and comfortable lives. Life that is based on the achievement of goals, money, and power, with the attendant pressures and constant competition, does not suit them. It is important to them that those around them not undermine their way of life and their personal goals, and that they feel that they are in control of their lives, and are free to decide for themselves how they want to live. They must be able to express themselves freely, and change any situation that does not appeal to them.

Health, growth, and development

People of the green type are powerfully kinesthetic (they have a sense of movement) and are strongly connected to their physical body. For them, body and mind are one inextricable unit: everything that affects the mind immediately affects the body, and vice versa. When they do not express - mainly verbally - their feelings, this is liable to manifest itself in bodily sensations ranging from discomfort to a full-blown disease.

In order for people of the green type to find harmony in their lives, they must take responsibility for their lives, create a link with their bodies and minds, and discern the natural flow of love and growth that exists both in the universe and in them.

When they recognize their goals and desires, they are granted nature's full support to realize them. Since they are natural healers, with a unique channeling ability, they have to acknowledge their goal in life. They are gifted with the exceptional ability to join body and mind, and to convey messages of friendship, love, and goodness of heart to the rest of mankind.

People of this type must be aware and in tune with their general feeling of love for life. When they do this, they find the inner strength to make the changes they themselves need, they understand and comprehend the changes that occur in their lives - they discover their true goals, which give flavor to their lives. When they allow their bodies and minds to behave naturally, they find the correct ways to fill up with energy and to store a great deal of energetic strength.

Because they understand their bodies, these people are generally very healthy - as along as they listen to their bodies, which guide them as to what is right and what is not, and how to balance and improve their health.

People of this type must remember the close link between them and nature, and not ignore their need for comfortable, quiet, and tranquil surroundings. They need a lot of time to themselves, and they derive a great deal of energy from spending a quiet and relaxing time in nature, or in a pleasant and comfortable home.

They must remember that sitting and having a calm and pleasant conversation with friends or family members, as well as enjoying nature in an enjoyable and relaxed way, are the type of things that fill them with positive energy, and help them maintain their equilibrium.

As we said before, people of the green type have an urgent and vital need to discuss their emotions and to communicate with their environment. They must remember this when their equilibrium fails, and they shut themselves up at home with the family pets. A good conversation with a close friend or family member, or a walk outdoors with a few friends, will improve their state and help to restore their equilibrium.

Neither fleeing from coping nor isolation and withdrawal is helpful to them.

When their emotions are blocked and their need to talk and express themselves - in whatever manner - is repressed, their health and mental state are harmed to a great extent. A simple, harmonious, and natural life is the life that is most suitable for people of this type. This is also the message that they can deliver to the world in which we live, which is moving dangerously far away from simplicity, the natural way, harmony, and nature. As teachers and care-gives, they certainly know how to impart these important insights to people. Helping others - as well as conveying this knowledge in any possible way - gives them the most wonderful and satisfying feeling imaginable.

Green, the color of these people, is the color of growth and development. When they do not fear change that results from growth, they may well find that nature supports every step they take.

The dark green personality type - the organizer

People of the dark green type are assertive (but conservative), determined, effective, stable, and stubborn. All told, they have impressive personalities. They closely resemble people of the green type in character; the main difference between them lies in the intensity, directness, and greater power of the dark green types.

Like people of the green type, these people are incredibly communicative, love nature and are close to it, enjoy abundance, prosperity, and luxury, and love to talk. However, they are far more ambitious than the green types, and more organized in their thoughts and *modus operandi*. Their way of thinking is quicker, more brilliant, and more dynamic than that of the green types. The dark green types stand out in society for their vitality, their superb intelligence, their excellent communicative ability, and their tendency to be surrounded by people and friends. While they prefer financial abundance and luxury, they also love a close bond to nature. People of this type, like those of the green type, represent the balance between body and mind.

People of this type are also wonderful conversationalists, and a good conversation about any topic under the sun - especially business, or things that will promote and enrich their personal development - is one of their favorite things. They need to be surrounded by people, and to express themselves verbally; this makes them feel balanced and full of life and energy. They are also blessed with the ability to capture the interest of their fellow conversationalists, mainly because of their directness and their superb, lucid intellect, and because of their appearance and personality, which impress the people around them from the outset.

When you come across one of these types, you may be surprised at how quickly and directly he expresses his opinion, even about your personal affairs, and you may not like the way in which he tells you exactly what you have to do in order to extricate yourself from some sticky situation, or how to solve a problem. Sometimes people of this type give their fellow conversationalist the feeling that they think they know everything better than anyone else - but to tell the truth, if you follow their advice, chances are that you will discover that it was precisely the right advice at the right time!

People of this type have the ability to get right to the heart of the problem, and to explain clearly and succinctly how to solve it. They do not get embroiled in lengthy explanations, and do not require a lot of time to understand anything. Their minds are so quick and incisive that they can summarize an entire conversation in a few accurate and clear sentences, while emphasizing the main points of the conversation.

People of this type are very competitive, ambitious, and quick-thinking. They require constant interest in their lives - on the conjugal level, in company, and in their occupations - and become bored easily in the absence of significant stimuli. They need intellectual growth and development, and constantly aspire to increase and enrich their knowledge. It is difficult for them to wind down and empty their minds because they are processing data and using their minds incessantly. Sometimes, their quickness of thought is liable to make them intolerant of others who are not quite as fast at processing intellectual data as they are.

They feel that their lives are full when they know exactly what tasks and aspirations lie before them. They measure a task according to the question of how fast and effectively it can be accomplished, and how great the chances are of them accomplishing it perfectly. Sometimes, after they have succeeded in realizing their aspirations, they may feel a kind of emptiness that makes them rush to find the next task to accomplish. For this reason, their lives are constantly filled with action.

Similar to people of the green type, the dark green types

are also occasionally inclined to fear change in their lifestyles, behavior, and way of thinking. They create their own world view and solid and precise opinions, and it is sometimes difficult for them to listen to or accept other views and opinions. Moreover, they do not like being told what to do and how to do it, and feel a great need to be independent and do things in their own way.

Occasionally, they feel a certain superiority vis-a-vis the rest of mankind, and this feeling makes it even harder for them to accept advice or orders from others, since people of the dark green type are certain that they can do everything better than anyone else.

They are perfectionists with high expectations of themselves and of others, to the point that they make life difficult for those around them. Sometimes, they set extremely high goals for themselves, and will not relax or feel satisfied until they have accomplished them perfectly. Their friends, family, and workers sometimes get the feeling that no matter how hard they try and how much they succeed in accomplishing the task or achieving the goal, their dark green friend will always find fault or have something to say - a critical comment that expresses a general attitude of "It could have been done better," or "I would have done it better."

People of this type must understand that if they learn to lower the level of their expectations of themselves and of others slightly, they will achieve the coveted feeling of satisfaction at the sight of an accomplished goal or a completed project more often and more easily.

Health, growth, and development

People of the dark green type have an extremely significant need to control their lives, both physically and mentally. They must keep this "need" in a state of balance. When they learn to look inward at their emotions, take full responsibility for their lives, and establish their life goals, they will feel balanced and harmonious. They must know how to plan their steps one at a time, and aim at a goal; in this way, their wishes will come true.

They must remember that they are linked and joined to the heart chakra, whose green color they represent, and the more they learn to open their hearts and work on becoming tolerant and patient, acknowledging the difference between people, and accepting people as they are, the greater the balance they will achieve.

They must be aware of their abilities - both physical and mental - and their expectations of themselves, all the while looking and checking to see if they are projecting their expectations onto the people close to them, both in their interpersonal relationships and in the professional framework. They must refrain from this behavior and attitude as a result of understanding themselves and of awareness. When they are in tune with their emotions and hearts, people of this type will find the way to channel their very powerful energies into positive and beneficial goals, and will feel more fulfilled. Moreover, their self-esteem will increase. When they look inside themselves, they may well discover that the strong will power they radiate, the power, and sometimes the domination, are nothing but a cover-up for genuine feelings and for the fear of failure, lack of esteem, and the feeling that they are not good enough, or "not as good as everyone else."

These feelings have to be dealt with radically, and not by attempting to impress or control their way of life or that of the people around them. Saying positive mantras that raise self-esteem, and looking into themselves in order to discover the true value of their personalities will help them to accept change and the unexpected in their lives, as well as other people's characters. They must accept and understand that their lack of confidence is not negative, and does not attest to a lack of inner power or to a personality defect, but rather is natural, accepted, and a part of life.

Similar to people of the green type, these people also need to internalize the knowledge that life is constant change, development, and growth; these aspects of life are natural and essential, and there is no need to fear them or try to control them. When they learn to accept themselves as they are, without aspiring to constant perfection, and learn to wind down and relax both physically and mentally, they will feel a great deal of relief in all facets of life, and much more energetic and liberated.

The blue personality type - the helper

You will identify the blue type when you observe him shedding sentimental tears during a movie such as "Lassie Come Home," as he rocks the baby in its cradle, alert and loving. When you tell him about a crisis you went through, or about a happy event in your life, you can see how he identifies with you by looking in his eyes and seeing how they shine when hearing about the happiness in your life, or when he offers you - as naturally as can be - a broad and soft shoulder to cry on when things are not as they should be.

People of the blue type came into the world in order to help mankind accept love, affection, and attention. Of all the color types, they are the ones who are the most supportive, caring, protective, and happy to help. Their aim in life is to serve, help, love, and give to others, and they live their lives through their hearts and emotions.

By means of their personalities, lives, and ways, they teach that without love, nothing in this world is worth anything. People of this type are sincere, decent, and moral, and believe in the values of tradition and in preserving values. They are big-hearted, friendly, extrovert, and warm. They operate mainly according to their emotions and intuition, and do not consider "realistic" facts to be exclusive truths. They have the inner knowledge, the wisdom, and the ability to know what's right without needing information or facts. When they listen to themselves, and are in tune with their inner voice, they know exactly what to do, and how and when to do it.

They have an amazing aptitude to make friends with other people, and sense their feelings as well as what is happening in their hearts very accurately. People of this type are the most sentimental of all the color types, and represent a fathomless well of emotions. They are so solicitous about other people that they sometimes care more about the people around them than about themselves.

They are born "care-givers" and parents; they always remember to take care of and support their nearest and dearest, the sick, and the less fortunate, never forget birthdays, and always offer a shoulder to cry on. They always advise, support, guide, and take care of others willingly and naturally. Love and their ability to accept and grant forgiveness are wonderful qualities that make blue types special and make other people feel fantastic in their company.

People of this type, whose color is reminiscent of the blue of the sea and water, express their feelings a lot through their eyes, which fill with tears and cry easily - as a reaction to sadness, joy, emotion, or anger. They are astoundingly empathetic, forgive and excuse easily, and are blessed with the wonderful quality of being able to bestow unconditional love. Sometimes, unfortunately, these marvelous qualities cause insensitive people to take advantage of them.

People of this type have no difficulty accepting the authority of others, and obey every order or demand naturally and unresistingly. Sometimes, in this way, they hand over the reins of their lives to other people, thus exposing themselves to being exploited or used, and consequently getting into painful and frustrating situations. Sometimes they feel that they are not in control of their lives, and that they are incapable of changing the situations in which they find themselves.

Another problem that arises with people of this type is excessive concern for other people, to the point of forgetting about themselves, and placing their own needs and desires at the bottom of their list of priorities. They sometimes spend so much time listening to and dealing with the problems of other people that they forget their own. They must always remember the importance of devoting time to their needs and to their physical, mental, and spiritual development, and know that they should spend more time on their personal growth.

People of this type foster a deep and real fear of rejection and emotional injury. For this reason, they are afraid of setting limits for others and saying "No" when it is necessary, because of the fear that they will be loved less or rejected. They tend to see the reflection of their fears in their fellow-man, and are therefore always afraid that others want to reject them or hurt them in some way. People of this type must understand that setting limits or saying "No" is not the same as saying "I don't love you," and it is the necessary and correct thing to do in many cases! When they are not aware of this, many blue types fall victim to the exploitation of other people, who take merciless advantage of their love and good-heartedness. People of this type must understand the importance of self-love, of self-esteem and recognition, and know how to actively set the correct limits - even for their friends, spouses, and children.

The problem of being unable to set limits is liable to be expressed in the energetic realm, too, when people deplete blue types of their strength and energy, and leave them exhausted. This exhaustion is also liable to stem from the way people of this type identify deeply with the problems and suffering of others. Sometimes, they identify with other people's pain and feel it so deeply that they begin to feel the suffering themselves, and are liable to identify with their fellow-man even to the point of "acquiring" a disease or a pain that is similar or identical to his. When they work as psychologists or healers, this problem is extremely significant, and they have to learn to set physical and mental limits, to reinforce their auras, and to perform energetic "protections" before the treatment, as well as energetic cleansing afterwards.

People of the blue type do not like physical activity and hard work. They sometimes feel that the outside world is too cold, aggressive, noisy, and insensitive. They prefer to live quietly in their emotional world, and they do not push themselves or aspire to win public acclaim, even though they sometimes do so because of their big contribution to society, and their participation in various organizations and occupations for the benefit of the public.

Health, growth, and development

In order to be healthy and balanced, people of this type must learn "self-love" - learn to accept, esteem, and love themselves, and not to expect this from others and live for the love of others. Because of their sensitivity and their profound emotions, they are liable to be easily hurt, and will sometimes do anything in order to gain attention and affection.

People of this type must understand that they are loved, and that love starts inside, within them. When they learn to love themselves, their strong fear of a lack of love and affection, and of abandonment and rejection, will gradually fade, giving way to sincere and genuine self-esteem and self-confidence, while they express their emotions and inner feelings freely, and enjoy lives filled with satisfaction, happiness, compassion, and love.

As we said before, it is extremely important for people of this type to know how to be assertive, to say "No" and to set limits when other people start to exploit their good-heartedness. When they finally decide to say "No" after their inner resistance to something crystallizes inside them, their inner strength increases, and as a result, their giving abilities, love, and compassion also increase and grow stronger.

People of this type must be aware of their emotional power and of the depth of their emotions. They have a sensitive and powerful emotional system, and the understanding of the link between their body and their mind will help them remain strong and healthy.

When they find themselves in a problematic situation, they must calm down, remain focused, and dive into their inner being. If they ask their question in a state of calmness and tranquillity, they will sense the answer immediately.

The challenge facing people of this type is not just to know how to listen to inner voices, but rather to trust them, and act and live according to them!

Since people of this type are capable of befriending and helping anyone (and we mean anyone!), they must make conscious decisions as to whom, of all the many people they know and support, they want to accept as friends. As close friends, they must choose people who are capable of returning love, and who know how to appreciate the love that people of the blue type give them in such enormous quantities!

It is important that they create a tranquil and harmonious environment for themselves, and devote time to themselves, in order to recharge their batteries. This is essential, since they often find themselves in situations of endless giving, and they have to learn to give to themselves as well. Listening to quiet and harmonious music, sitting quietly with a good and moving book, and tuning in to themselves, while allowing the quiet and the tranquillity to flow inside them, are important activities for people of this type - for the sake of achieving harmony and tranquillity, and in order to link up with their vocation in life.

For this reason, prayer and meditation are extremely significant to people of this type, in order to attain inner peace and inner happiness, link up to themselves, and recharge their batteries and energy. Joining groups that engage in quiet, tranquil spiritual activities such as meditation will bring people of this type into contact with people who are similar to them, and with people who appreciate their wonderful character and their giving nature.

In addition, it must be remembered that nurturing the spiritual dimension in the lives of people of this type gives them tremendous power, and helps them channel their special abilities toward the good of mankind.

The indigo personality type - the seeker

People of the indigo type are spiritual in every sense of the word. They live their lives through their inner emotions and profound feelings, and are permanently tuned into their inner knowledge, their intuition, and their upper self. Their lives are a long search for a higher truth and a loftier awareness. They radiate authenticity and clarity to an extent that is not found in any of the other color types. They are quiet and easy-going types, and have a very strong need to express their spirituality and their religiosity. Indigo types are independent, very creative, and brilliant.

This type often has a soft and sensitive - sometimes even androgynous - exterior, and his personality comprises both female and male aspects and elements. For that reason, as well as their highly developed spirituality, people are sometimes inclined to view them as unusual - and in extreme cases, as strange and eccentric.

Many of them are born as aware creatures, and as children already know what they want and how they have to conduct themselves. These types are aware of their inner truth, feel it, think about it - and act. They cannot be told how to behave, what to think, or in what to believe, because by means of their strong inner guidance, they are well aware of their inner truth. They have a sense of self-respect, and a system of unique beliefs and perceptions of their own. They are sincere and independent, very popular, and full of compassion for all human beings.

People of the indigo type live in order to feel life, as celestial and universal creatures, filled with love and compassion. Life for them is an infinite ocean of energy, love, compassion, and unlimited possibilities, and they feel a great deal of satisfaction if they can express their spiritual or religious feelings, knowing that the world around them reacts to their special message. People of this type see in love and in God the force that motivates and unites the world. They see people as celestial beings, far beyond the perception of body, emotion, and intellect, and linked to the upper force - they feel that the universe, all its components, and the superior force, are one, linked and united.

They cannot understand how people can harm one another, animals, and the universe, because they are well aware that every action that is performed by one person affects the whole of mankind.

These types are tremendously aware of the world and humanity, and constitute the leaders of the New Age. They do not need proof or information in order to understand that our world is in a situation that is far from positive - they feel it themselves - and they do not need a reason to help the spiritual growth of mankind.

In the past, people of this type would do their spiritual work in organized or religious groups. Nowadays, in a society in which the individual can do as he pleases, these types are no longer afraid of prejudices and religious persecution, and they are free to live in accordance with their basic feelings and their inner truth, and communicate with God in their own way.

People of this type are enlightened and aware when it comes to their perception of humanity and the universe, and are guided by intuition and their inner knowledge, as well as by higher sources of insight. They know that we are all divine creatures, that life is significant, and that we, human beings, create our own reality.

Health, growth, and development

As we have already mentioned, people of the indigo type must link up to their inner knowledge and their upper self. In order to maximize their strength, they must heed the inner voices that guide them. When they live in accordance with their beliefs, emotions, and intuition, they create an environment that radiates love, peace, and understanding.

People of this type have delicate and fragile bodies, and they are not accustomed to the environmental pressure and tension that are prevalent nowadays. Their unusual appearance and their indefinable (by the simplistic and sometimes ignorant definitions of society) behavior also make it difficult for them to adapt to our insensitive and unbalanced society. It is extremely important that people of this type create a quiet and balanced environment for themselves, one that will enable them to remain tranquil, focused on their spiritual work, and tuned into their inner knowledge.

When people of this type are in a state of harmony, they have no problem recharging their batteries by means of their spiritual work.

It is not surprising if they feel that the external world is too brutal, noisy, and raucous for them, since they are very sensitive to the obvious lack of balance in today's society. A quiet environment, which affords them constant spiritual development, together with several close and loving friends, peace, tranquillity, and harmony, enable this type of person to be in complete balance, and to link up to the energies of the universe. People of this type understand that they are part of the breathing and living organism that is called the universe, and that they are the children of God, and part of His breath.

It is very important that they be linked to their mission and their vision; meditation, prayer, and linking up to God and to their upper self will help them to accomplish their mission, and to achieve balance, power, and harmony. By linking up to their upper self and their inner guide, they will receive answers to all their questions. They will create harmony in their lives and in the whole world if they live their lives through awareness and the expression of their inner strength and beliefs - in love, compassion, and understanding.

The important mission, and the one that is not easy for people of this type, is to go out into the world and make their spiritual messages and beliefs heard, seen, and felt.

They have the ability to show people how a holistic and spiritual society will look, and when they do that, their contribution to humanity is enormous.

The purple personality type - the visionary

The color purple is the color of the sixth chakra - the third eye chakra - and also symbolizes the seventh chakra - the crown chakra. These two chakras symbolize a high state of awareness that is close to divine awareness and to the link with higher states of awareness and senses. For this reason, people of this type are considered to be visionaries, in every sense of the word.

People of the purple type have extremely strong personalities. They are charismatic, dynamic, and futuristic, and have lofty ideals. They have a vision of the future of the world, and entertain hopes for a better and more advanced world. Similar to the color purple, people of this type are blessed with both the blue and the red qualities, and those two colors together elevate them to a higher level of awareness.

Most people of this type feel that they have to do something of great significance in their lives, and indeed, their function is to lead mankind to a new age of prosperity and perfection. In order to perform this function, they are blessed with the physical, emotional, and intellectual strength, and superb intellectual and intuitive abilities that are prerequisites for effecting the changes both in their lives and in the lives of other people.

People of the purple type combine the qualities of the red color with those of the blue color in their personalities. For this reason, their lives have to combine the aspects of both types, at the same time raising them to a higher level of awareness.

They must combine the blue. qualities - intuition,

sensitivity, compassion, solicitude, and love - with the red qualities - physical power, strength, activity, and passion.

In general, people of this type have a strong body and a powerful energetic ability. They have to release their pent-up physical energy by engaging in physical activity and sports. Similar to people of the red type, calmness induced by action - that is, creative physical activity that engenders calmness - is their most suitable way of releasing surplus physical and mental energy.

Sometimes, these types are liable to appear cold and distant, but this is not the case. Deep inside, they are sensitive, emotional, and full of passion. They have the passion of the color red, but also the sensitivity and the depth of emotion of the color blue, and that is why they are cautious with their emotions. Their aloof appearance occasionally serves as a defense for them, since their great sensitivity means that they are easily hurt.

Although other people view them as having a great deal of self-esteem, self-confidence, and power, people of this type sometimes suffer from a lack of inner confidence that cannot be detected by strangers. They have a strong perfectionist tendency, as well as a self-critical sense that sometimes causes them to feel worthless, and to have guilt feelings.

Even after they have completed a particular project successfully, people of this type are liable to look for the little errors, and feel that they could have done things better, more quickly, and more efficiently. Their hypercritical nature often causes them feelings of regret and dissatisfaction with the results of their work.

People of this type feel the need to express their vision by means of creation and invention, and their lives would seem worthless to them if they did not fulfill this need. They are extremely flexible by nature, and they view life as marvelous and magical. These people have charismatic and truly magnetic personalities. They have a great deal of emotional depth, and enchant the people around them. They believe in their ability to turn dreams into reality; as a result, it is in their power - with the help of superb mental and spiritual abilities - to realize their dreams. They feel the energies, can link up to them, and often have a clear view of the future. Their lives are a combination of apparent contradictions: objectivity and physical awareness together with strong and dominant mysticism.

People of the purple type are very independent, and need a lot of space and time to themselves. This can be seen in their preferred choice of residence - a space that is as big, open, and wide as possible, which can contain their forceful energy.

Life in a small, closed space in a small community is liable to cause them a great deal of suffering. They are eager to spread their vision throughout the entire world, and they cannot countenance being in a small, limited place for any length of time.

Health, growth, and development
One of the biggest and most important challenges facing people of the purple type is the need to develop confidence and belief in their intuition and inner guidance, and to follow their vision. If they learn to focus their energy, to believe in and trust their vision, and to keep their feet planted firmly on the ground, they can achieve anything. When they live their belief and vision enthusiastically, their hearts will always lead them along the path that is right for realizing them.

People of this type must be cognizant of their strong self-criticism and their sometimes exaggerated sense of perfectionism, get them into the correct proportion, and know how to pat themselves on the back without always getting into the minute details and seeing how they could have done things better and avoided minor errors. Things like this make life more difficult for them, and ultimately cause them to feel worthless. People of this type must know how to deal with feelings of guilt and worthlessness correctly, and let go of them, when necessary, so as not to be too hard on themselves.

Although people of this type consider regular conversations or socializing with friends to be a waste of time, preferring to focus on their creative or spiritual work, they must learn to loosen the reins slightly, to allow themselves to have a good time without pangs of conscience about "wasted time and lack of effectiveness," and to get out of their "cave" and enjoy life. They must learn to focus on their third eye, and stop their unbalanced pursuit of the realization of their vision. If they are in touch with their intuition, they will discover and realize their correct vocation in life anyway. People of this type must know that so long as they do not live their vision, and do not realize themselves, they will feel the inner tension and lack of peace of mind that stems from the non-realization of their vocation. Devoting time to themselves, focusing, and meditation will help them get in touch with their inner vision.

When people of this type link up to the universal energy via meditation, yoga, creation, and other things, they gain an unlimited supply of energy and abundance.

People of this type must remember that if they find their place and function in the universe, and feel the link to the great cosmic energy and the universe, the universe will support them unconditionally, and will accompany them every step of the way.

The lavender personality type - the dreamer

You can identify people of this type by their fragile exterior, their weak bodies, their pale skin, their "arty" look, and their appearance, which may well remind you of a fairy or an angel. When you go and speak to them, you will probably find that they are floating in another world. Indeed, people of the lavender type live in a kind of different reality, a world of fantasies and dreams, in which fairies and angels reign supreme, and where there are various myths and different and higher dimensions of reality. People of this type spend most of their time in the world of the imagination, sketching and spinning daydreams. Their brains are free to discover completely new possibilities, perceptions, and levels of reality.

No practical boundary will stop their train of thought - whatever they are capable of imagining is genuine and realistic for them. To them, the world of Alice in Wonderland seems perfectly possible. For that reason, their ideas are likely to be wonderfully novel, their thinking far-reaching, and their creativity astounding. Many of them can see and feel energies, other dimensions, or different levels of reality. Their bodies are extremely sensitive, and their inner senses are constantly active. This affords them access to spiritual and ethereal energies that they can use for healing.

People of this type have the ability to induce a state of

mind that is full of magic, imagination, and fantasy in the people around them. They are likely to be entertaining, amusing, and gratifying to those around them. When they are in a state of balance, they can be marvelous story-tellers, artists, and writers. By dint of their fertile and colorful imagination, they are able to describe and create enchanted, mysterious, and wonderful worlds that feature ghosts and fairies and beings from faraway worlds.

People of this type need unlimited freedom, without mental, physical, or spiritual boundaries. They are able to carry mankind beyond its borders and limitations, to a new and unknown world. They need perfect freedom to follow their imagination in any direction it wants to take them.

Their perception of the world is completely different than that of the rest of humanity, and they feel that their dreams and fantasies can create any reality that they desire. They are aware of the fact that our dreams, thoughts, imagination, and wishes actually create the physical reality in which we live. "First think, then act" is the most ancient law of the universe. The energy of our thoughts has the potential to become a physical reality (and whoever doesn't believe this should try it out for himself!). People of the lavender type understand this ancient law very well, and can use their thoughts and imagination to change physical reality.

People of the lavender type are not blessed with a strong physical body, and physical reality, as most people perceive it, seems cold, harsh, and even brutal to them. They look for environments and situations in which life is easy, slow-flowing, beautiful, and enchanted. Since they live mainly in their inner worlds and imagination, they do not like to confront the reality of the material world.

Health, growth, and development

In order to remain balanced and harmonious, people of the lavender type must learn to "land their spaceships" every now and then, take their heads out of the clouds, and feel the earth under their feet...

These types must understand that there is a reason why we live in this three-dimensional world. We came into a world in which matter is real and tangible, and in which we have a physical body and physical needs. While it is true that coping with material reality is not easy for people of this type, they nevertheless have to look inside themselves and find the courage to remain with their feet planted on the ground, while their heads are in the clouds, because they are able to link fantasy and reality, and turn thought and imagination into matter, which is a special and marvelous ability. This ability could be beneficial and advantageous to mankind as well as enchant the human race if people of this type were wise enough to remain linked to their surroundings and to the outside world, and utilize their creativity and imagination for the good and happiness of all people.

Fighting these marvelous qualities of imagination and fantasy is futile. Just like most people need sleep in order to function normally, so people of this type require serenity and entry into the world of imagination and fantasy in order to feel balanced and harmonious. But they have to create the suitable and correct environment and time for themselves in addition to balancing the world of the imagination and the material world. Coping with their weaknesses - instead of detaching themselves from the world by running away and hiding - will enable them to discover their inner strength, to express themselves, and to express their creativity and strength. The more they succeed in grounding themselves and keeping both feet on the ground, the more they will succeed in turning their ideas and fantasies into reality.

Since they spend most of their time in the world of the imagination, in which material laws are not valid, people of this type are inclined to lose touch with their bodies. They constantly have to remember that we are human creatures who consist of a number of dimensions, and that the material dimension is one of them. They must make sure to take care of their bodies on a daily basis. A healthy life, including activities that create a link with the earth, such as gardening, agriculture, swimming, and hiking, can strengthen and balance these people's link to reality.

The white personality type - the enlightened

The color white symbolizes the highest vibration of energy, the universal life force, and divine energy. White light itself is not color, but rather a combination of all the colors of the spectrum. In this way, people of the white type are the embodiment of unadulterated spirituality. People of this type are exceptionally spiritual. They are linked and joined to the divine, and guided by their upper self. Their vocation is to teach humanity that the "electro-magnetic" is situated everywhere and in everything, and that human beings are entities that are full of power and spirituality. People of this type feel that they are channels for the flow of divine abundance, for healing, and for stimulating the divine breath in people (that is, they often function as pipelines for channeling).

People of this type are quiet and modest, and although

they may have a great deal of knowledge, do not tend to flaunt it. Their main motive in this world, according to which they measure the degree of their "success," is the extent of their link to the source of divine energy, inner clarity, and the extent of their ability to receive and convey healing energy using their bodies as pipelines. They see life in all its vibrations as a sight that reflects their spiritual state and their level of spiritual development, and the extent to which they succeed in conveying and applying the energy of light in their lives. The purpose of their life is linking up to the celestial, to the light, and to divine love.

People of this type have an admirable ability to be objective. When they are in a situation that demands action and solutions - in their daily lives as well - they can put their thoughts and emotions aside so as not to disrupt their ability to see things as they are. Their pure personalities are reminiscent of a prism in which the light is reflected; the purer and more linked up they are, the greater the amount of light that is reflected in them and passes through them. Their awareness is the most powerful tool they possess, and with its help, they can work wonders. They are well aware of being multi-dimensional souls that have experienced - or are experiencing - events in different times and dimensions than the ones in this world. They can link up to different states of awareness and to deeper levels of inner awareness, all the while perceiving the material world as only one of many dimensions in which there are limitations and boundaries that do not exist in other dimensions. They know how to discern the illusions and limitations of this world, and rise above them in their awareness.

Similar to the color white, which comprises all the colors of the spectrum, so people of the white type contain the qualities of all the colors inside them. They can "switch skins" and easily adopt other behavior and thought patterns. They can easily tune in to other people. When they are in an unbalanced state, and are not properly linked to their inner side and to their motivating energy, they are able to take on the characteristics and the patterns of behavior, thought, and emotions of other people. Sometimes they are unaware of the fact that they suddenly begin to speak and behave like their fellow-conversationalist, to feel his emotions, and even to read his thoughts. In a balanced state of awareness, they can use this special ability to heal and understand other people as well as themselves. As practitioners, this ability gives them a tremendous advantage and is of great help in healing and therapy.

In an unbalanced state, people of this type are liable to attract the energies of other people to themselves, which can cause them to receive negative and unclean energies from other people, or to unconsciously draw out other people's positive energies, thus causing them harm.

People of the white type greatly enjoy reading books, seeing movies and shows, and visiting exhibitions. The link to creation, as well as the new and fascinating information that reaches them via these media enriches and edifies them greatly. They are able to get to the bottom of things and discover their hidden aspects easily. They do not like crowded places, and need a lot of time to themselves in order to cut off energetically, recharge their energy, and look inside themselves through meditation, techniques of balance and expanding, and personal and spiritual ceremonies. For this reason, they often determine a particular time for going off and isolating themselves, and for withdrawing into themselves and spiritual learning.

People of this type need beautiful, clean, pleasant, and quiet surroundings. They love to create such an environment for themselves, since it is compatible with their spiritual development and is a pleasant and comfortable place within which they can charge themselves energetically. They try as much as possible to get away from noisy, dirty, unpleasant places, as well as from harsh, noisy, and insensitive company. Any stressful disturbances - big or small, physical, emotional, or intellectual - are difficult for people of this type to bear, because they do not know how to cope with them, and feel that they are disrupting their inner balance.

Health, growth, and development

In order to be balanced, healthy, and harmonious, people of the white type must be linked to their life's purpose. An aware way of life of the soul, understanding that human beings are here, in the material world, only for a short time, in order to carry out the repairs and do the jobs that they were destined to do in the physical world - constantly linked to cosmic energy - is the suitable and correct way of life for people of this type. In order to be a clean and powerful pipeline for the exalted cosmic energy that passes through them, people of this type have to see that they live in a tranquil, quiet, clean, and pure environment. Devoting time to nurturing their home environment, surrounding themselves with crystals, flowers, and plants, or spending time in natural surroundings, is essential for the continuation of their spiritual development and their personal growth. They have to understand that the extremely powerful energy that passes through them requires that they be a clean and obstacle-free channel. For this reason, they must take care of their bodies and their health. The stronger, cleaner, and purer their body, soul, and spirit are, the more divine light will pass through them, and their healing powers and energy will increase.

They must ensure that they eat correctly, engage in healthful physical activity, and spend time in the bosom of nature, or on the seashore. Of course, food colorings, preservatives, cigarettes, alcohol, and an unbalanced diet have a bad effect on everyone, regardless of color type. Since the balance of people of this type depends on the level of their ability to serve as a channel for divine energy, refraining from ingesting these dangerous and toxic substances is more significant and pertinent with regard to them than any to other color type.

People of this type must be aware of their ability to pick up energies from other people. It is important for them to be strong and focused in their interaction with those around in order not to "draw" energies from them, or absorb negative energies from other people. Because their souls are so pure and white, any speck that sticks to them is immediately noticeable, and affects them and their balance - in the same way that a stain, even a single one, on an item of white clothing is glaringly conspicuous. After being in the company of many people, or people whose energy is not very familiar to them, they must take note whether they attracted certain inappropriate energy to themselves, and cleanse and purify themselves of it.

Of course, people of this type must find, learn, or develop ways of linking up to the light and to the universal energy. Various forms of meditation, focusing on the link to the divine light, and living in a state of awareness of the soul (that is, when the person is aware of the soul within him, of its desires and needs - love, light, compassion, a link to the divine, giving and so on - and operates according to those needs in his daily life), will help people of this type to remain on the correct path to fulfilling their vocation in this world. Moreover, people of this type must remember - something that they probably know well - that their powers were given to them in order to help, advance, and enlighten mankind. They have to allow and permit themselves to share the wonderful light that crosses their path, and be aware of that fact every moment of their lives.

People of this type are familiar with the power of thought, whose aim is (for all of us) to heal and to benefit other people. Because of their ability to link up easily and immediately to higher energies, when they send thoughts of love, healing, and blessing - to friends, relatives, and even to people who did not treat them well, or caused them anguish - they have the ability to effect a change in the lives and development of these people, and at the same time, reinforce their strength, their spiritual development, and their ability to receive ever-increasing amounts of divine light.

PART 3

The Shape of the Aura

Now that we have dealt with the colors of the aura, we have to relate to an additional factor that affects the aura and is important in its diagnosis: the shape of the aura. The shape of the electro-magnetic field that surrounds the body reveals many details about the personality of the person, and reveals his basic tendencies.

The shape of the aura, from the point of view of height and width, differs from person to person. Even in a particular person, there are likely to be periods in which the aura is bigger and broader, or smaller and narrower.

In general, the clearer and bigger the shape of the aura, and the stronger and more vivid its colors, the greater its energetic level. However, people who have only started trying to see the aura, and who are not yet experienced, must take into account the possibility that they are not seeing the entire range of the aura.

Experts in seeing auras agree on the following characteristics:

An electro-magnetic field that is very close to the body may attest to inward withdrawal, to strong introversion, and to a great deal of restraint, especially if the color blue is conspicuous in the field of the aura.

A broad electro-magnetic field (at a distance from the body) generally indicates strong energy, activity, and extroversion.

A small electro-magnetic field may also indicate introversion, but in addition, it may well attest to fatigue, to a kind of weakness, or to concentrated activity that does not spread outward.

An especially large electro-magnetic field may be

indicative of a great deal of energy, extroversion, and power, especially of the spiritual kind. (Nevertheless, it is, of course, very important to analyze the colors of the aura, too!)

If the electro-magnetic field is "cloudy" or "misty," or there are dots of color in, it is generally an indication of tension and pressure.

Pale, dull, faded, or very dark colors, and most especially holes and hollows, may be indicative of a significant lack of energy.

If there is a concentration of a great deal of energy around a particular energy center (chakra), or around a particular body part, this attests to excessive activity or to a lot of activity in this center or area.

A relatively small amount of energy around a particular area of the body or around a particular energy center (chakra) is generally caused by tension and problems in the region, and leads to an uneven and non-flowing passage of energy.

If there is a lot of energy around a particular energy center (chakra), this could be an indication of its excellent abilities, and of the fact that a lot of attention is paid to it.

Of course, the analysis is not that simple. We have to take into account various components of the structure, shape, and colors of the aura, as well as the concentrations of color and energies around particular chakras.

For instance, a large amount of energy around the sixth (third eye) chakra may attest to a person who devotes a lot of time to spiritual development, meditation, and awareness. On the other hand, however, in an unbalanced state, it could attest to "floating," or to detachment from or a lack of reality.

Every one of the states can be interpreted either way, and the entire picture must be examined. In the above case, it is very important to scrutinize the base chakra according to its manifestation in the aura.

If, for example, the base chakra is active in a harmonious way, this will be revealed in the fact that the person's link to the earth is balanced. If there is some kind of lack or imbalance in the base chakra, there are more grounds for the interpretation of disharmony caused by excessive activity around the third eye chakra.

Although the shape of the aura changes according to the general condition of the person, and to his condition at the given time, it is possible to see that the general shape usually remains the same (or characterizes the person in most cases).

When we set about analyzing the appearance of the aura, there are five primary parameters to which we relate:

1. The energies of the left side of the body:

The left side of the body is activated physically by the right hemisphere of the brain. The right hemisphere of the brain is responsible for intuition, imagination, and creativity. The left side of the body symbolizes the feminine, passive, introvert pole.

The color of the aura that is seen on its left side represents the frequency of the energy that flows into the person's energy field. It shows the quality of the energy that the person receives and absorbs, energy that is significant vis-a-vis the person's future. The colors on the left side of the person's body clearly reflect the person's condition, and attest mainly to his emotional and intuitive state.

2. The energies of the right side of the body:

The right side of the body is activated by the left hemisphere of the brain. The left hemisphere of the brain is responsible for reason, logic, organization, and verbal skills. The right side of the body symbolizes the masculine, active, extrovert pole.

The color of the aura that is seen on its right side represents the person's attitude toward life, and what he is transmitting and giving at this moment. This is the energy that is transmitted to the environment, and is felt and received by the people around him. The state of the energies on this side also attests to the state of the person from the intellectual and analytical points of view.

3. The energy of the head:

The energy above the head represents the person's path and way of thinking, as well as what is happening to him at this moment. By observing this energy, it is easy to know if the person is thinking positive or negative thoughts.

4. The energy of the heart:

The energy of the heart teaches us how the person copes with his emotions. It is indicative of the person's ability to love and cope with love, and of the way in which he copes with, receives, and expresses his inner feelings. In addition, it also provides a certain indication of the person's physical immunity, the action of his immune system, and his resistance to disease.

5. The energy of the throat:

The energy of the throat attests to the person's communicative abilities and modes, to his creativity, and to the expression of his creativity. The appearance of dark shadows, hollows, holes, or "clouds" in this area - or an especially small aura - attest to communicative or creative blockages, to problems of self-expression (that can be physical, such as stuttering, as well as emotional, such as the inability to express himself in public, or to express his thoughts clearly), and to problems with communicating correctly with his surroundings.

In the following sections, we will learn how to strengthen the energy around these centers, and in the chapter on cleansing and purifying the aura, we will learn how to clean the "mists" and dark "clouds" that are found around the energy centers and the entire aura.

It must be remembered that even people who do not have the ability to see or feel the aura must ensure that they strengthen it, reinforce its power, and cleanse it.

Strengthening, cleansing, and protecting the electro-magnetic field

As we mentioned previously, our aura is in a state of constant change, and is affected by many different factors. Emotional states and mental attitudes, as well as physical states, all exert a great effect on the aura. In Kirlian photography, it is possible to see how the aura is affected by the content and type of thoughts that emanate from the mental body, from the emotions that are expressed in the emotional body, and from the state of vitality of the etheric body and the physical body. It is astonishing to see in a Kirlian photograph how negative thoughts have a "blocking" effect that creates blockages on the surface of the aura, while positive thoughts have a "strengthening" and empowering (balancing) effect on the electro-magnetic field. It can be seen that when we are speaking about a topic that affects us mentally and emotionally, the aura changes in accordance with the content that is being discussed and felt.

There are many different factors that affect the electro-magnetic field, and they can be divided into two groups: **internal factors** and **external factors**.

Internal factors are within our control - directly - even if people do not always think that this is the case.

External factors - amazingly - are also partially within our control, but the control requires much more practice and spiritual work (and, of course, control of the internal factors).

There are many interrelated internal factors that affect the aura, its colors, its strength, its cleanliness, and its power. In other words, an aura that gets "dirty" is liable to get weaker, and to lose more and more of its power. It should be understood that the aura constitutes an electro-magnetic field that protects the body, and it has the ability to filter out harmful vibrations. The aura's filtering ability depends on its cleanliness and power. The weaker its filtering ability, the greater the person's susceptibility to negative and harmful external influences. The weaker the aura, the weaker and more vulnerable the person's body, nervous system, and emotional and mental state.

The internal factors that weaken the aura can be divided into several groups:

The first group includes factors that weaken the aura as a result of the weakening of the body and injury to it, when the first aura to be harmed will probably be the aura of the physical body. (Remember, however, that there are no hard and fast rules about this.) These factors include smoking, incorrect nutrition, alcohol consumption, a lack of sleep and rest, tension and stress, exaggerated and exhausting work, a lack of physical activity, and other factors of this kind.

The second group includes negative emotions. These weaken the aura very significantly, and are liable to cause serious damage over the long term. These emotions include anger, depression, nervousness, aggressiveness, belligerence, frustration, a lack of a suitable outlet for venting emotions, guilt feelings, self-castigation, jealousy and envy, feelings of inferiority, feelings of deprivation, and so on. This group also includes residual subconscious traumas and negative emotions from the past.

The third group consists of the factors that weaken the aura via the thought aura. (It must be remembered that all the layers of the aura affect and are affected by one another.) This group includes negative thoughts and beliefs: negative thoughts about oneself, such as "I won't succeed,"

"I'm not good enough," "I'm not clever enough," and so on; negative thoughts and beliefs about the world, such as "All women are the same," "Money doesn't grow on trees," "Life is difficult and dangerous," "No one loves me," and so on. This group also includes the different attitudes toward life, such as a non-flowing attitude, a lack of happiness, a lack of faith, excessive skepticism, and the like.

The fourth group includes the factors that weaken the aura as a result of an injury to it (the aura of the person himself or someone else's aura - a person, an animal, or a plant), and the apparent rejection of the good that is offered by the universal forces. This group includes all the "mistakes" in human interaction and relationships - a disparaging attitude toward people, animals, and plants, impatience, intolerance, the use of dirty words, insults (an insult, for instance, is liable to weaken the auras of both the victim and the person who is doing the insulting!), immoral acts, a non-caring attitude, not listening to others, excessive self-absorption, and other factors.

It is very easy to identify and sense the **external factors**. When a person sits at a computer for hours on end, he is liable to feel weak or dizzy afterwards.

When a person enters a room in which an argument or quarrel is raging, he is liable to sense the negative vibrations that are present and that reach his aura.

These external factors include radiation - the radiation from computers, TV sets, microwave ovens, cellular phones, and so on, an extreme lack of cleanliness and tidiness, the use of chemicals, fruits and vegetables that have been sprayed with pesticides, low-quality food that contains artificial preservatives, air pollution, constant loud noise, high-decibel and aggressive music, a lot of artificial light, and being in the presence of a person with negative energies - a person who is nervous, aggressive, or an "energy-drainer" (the kind of person who is extremely tiresome; after being in his company, you feel fatigued, debilitated, and drained of energy). Moreover, quarrels and rows have a harmful effect, as do jealousy and envy, being in places where the energy is not clean - such as hospitals or places where serious events (from the point of view of energy) have occurred, a stressful environment, and so on.

Naturally, it is preferable to distance oneself from all these harmful factors. It does not mean, of course, that we have to refrain from visiting a friend in the hospital, but rather that we have to know that it is necessary to strengthen our auras (first of all, by not letting them become weak as a result of factors that we can control!), and we have to know how to cleanse them of the non-positive energies that are liable to adhere to them. Some of these factors are not very easy to change, but, surprisingly enough, it is the factors that we can control that have the greatest effect on the aura.

A person who can teach himself not to lose energy as a result of anger is also likely, at a certain point, to learn how to safeguard his energy in the presence of angry people, and how to avoid harming it.

There is no need to utilize far-reaching techniques - all that needs to be done is to recognize the negativity of these factors, and to try and avoid negative emotional factors: not to get angry, to try and make oneself happy during sad times, not to get caught up in self-pity, and so on.

Strengthening the thought (mental) aura

As we stated previously, strengthening the mental aura may change a person's life drastically. He may find himself moving from a distressing, saddening, and stressful life environment to a better, more pleasant, and healthier one - even on the economic level - just by changing his thought patterns! This fact, which sounds contrived to many people, is a clear and existing fact. To tell the truth, I have not yet met a person who worked seriously on changing his thought patterns and did not experience an extreme and satisfying change in his life.

One of the ways in which it is possible to work on the mental aura is by identifying defective thought patterns and negative beliefs. It is possible to take any sphere of life in which the person feels "stuck" and unsatisfied, and examine the person's "inner" attitude toward that sphere.

For instance, if there are problems in the interpersonal realm - the person feels that no matter where he is, he encounters difficult, uncompromising, and uncaring people - he must examine his set of beliefs regarding the world. It is possible that he believes the world to be a difficult and dangerous place, where dog eats dog. This negative belief must be changed. One of the ways of doing so is by preparing and internalizing aphorisms that contain positive thoughts. For example, "The world is a pleasant place to live in; I am surrounded by good and loving people," or "I live in perfect harmony with my surroundings." This must be repeated as many times as possible during the day - at least thirty times a day for three weeks - to start with.

It is astounding to discover that after accumulating

experience for a long time in identifying and changing thought patterns, the power of thought is strengthened to the point that the defective thought pattern may well disappear within a very short time, and with it the unpleasant situation (in the same way as working on our leg muscles for a certain length of time will bring us to the point that we can run much faster).

An additional method that is incredibly effective is dividing a sheet of paper into two columns - one entitled "Thought Column," and the other "Reaction Column." In the first column, the person writes the positive thought, such as "I love and esteem myself." In the second column, he writes his reaction, for example, "It is difficult for me to believe that." The reaction can range from feelings of disbelief in what is written, of "feeling stupid," and of nervousness, to physical symptoms starting with various pains and ending with a sudden need to release and empty oneself. In this method, the positive thought pattern is internalized, and the negative pattern of thought or its various expressions is expelled.

When a positive thought pattern is internalized, it must be remembered that we are "talking" to the subconscious. The subconscious listens to everything that is said to it without filtering, separating, or interpreting. Therefore, if the person says to himself, "I am not afraid to drive," for instance, there is every chance that his subconscious will pick up the word "afraid," and the words "to drive." When it joins the words together, it may well pick up a fear of driving. For this reason, positive words must be used when creating the sentences containing positive thoughts, such as "I feel confident and safe when I drive."

One of my patients, a young woman in general good health, complained that every time she went out for a social encounter, to school, to her crafts class, or to her treatment with me, she suffered from severe, almost paralyzing pains in her legs, even though she did not have a long way to walk. At home, the pains disappeared quickly. She did not suffer from any physical problem. Since she thought that perhaps her shoes were causing the pains, she bought expensive and comfortable orthopedic shoes - to no avail, however.

I asked her to select one of the following positive-thinking sentences: "I am free to come and go as I please," "I walk peacefully and safely through life," "My legs carry me everywhere comfortably and lightly." She had to write the sentence in the "Thought Column" every day, and in the "Reaction Column."

Since she felt that the sentence, "I walk peacefully and safely through life," suited her best, she chose it, and wrote it three times a day, while listening to and being very aware of the various different feelings that it invoked in her - among them also memories of her childhood. She also recited the sentence during the day while doing the daily household chores. Two weeks later, the pains in her legs were a thing of the past, and the patient had a clear insight as to why they had occurred at all.

People who have the ability to see and sense the aura can see how, when someone speaks about a certain subject, or is in the middle of a discussion or argument, his thoughts are not actually focused on the subject, but rather stray to another matter - generally an emotional one - and veer off the path in order to deal with that particular emotional problem. In cases such as these, the awareness is not focused on the body, and loses itself in past emotions.

When this is brought to the speaker's attention, it frequently transpires that he is not in the least aware of the process that is occurring within him.

A similar thing may happen in the mental sphere. When conscious thought is not anchored in the body, the attention may be diverted to old thought patterns. For instance, when a girl tells her friend, who suffers from "chronic" problems with men, about her new boyfriend, her "single" friend's old thought patterns are likely to kick in immediately, and thought patterns such as "I'll never find the love of my life" or "I don't deserve love" surface, form the root of her unconscious resistance to what her friend is saying, and are liable to spark an unconscious conflict between the two.

A common problem with many people - perhaps even the majority of people - is the difficulty in remaining focused on a particular thing for a relatively long period of time, without irrelevant emotional and thought patterns surfacing and disrupting the course of the interaction or the deed. Techniques and activities for focusing the thoughts, for emptying oneself of emotions and thoughts - such as meditation or conscious focusing on a particular object or deed - help maintain concentration and the state of awareness, thereby helping maintain the aura's state of balance.

A person who has developed a higher state of awareness knows how to identify the situations in which his attention and concentration stray from the main topic, and does not allow them to wander. Maintaining concentration causes his aura to resonate and vibrate harmoniously, and to affect the environment harmoniously and positively.

It is important to know that every disturbance that occurs in our electro-magnetic field unconsciously affects other people as well as our entire surroundings. This matter is extremely important. Unclean, "confused" thoughts mixed with irrelevant emotions and entangled in old thought and emotional patterns affect the entire interaction of the person with his surroundings, starting with his interpersonal relationships and his career, and ending with the effect on the entire world. This is no exaggeration.

It can be seen that the awareness of many people is focused on money, power, and sex - or on spiritual development, ecology, and social balance. It is possible to see the above mentioned dominant topics everywhere, and their strong influence on the various media.

This is an illustration of a thought pattern and an emotional pattern that resonate in many people, become more and more dominant, and affect and take control of the world.

This form of self-interested, unclean, and pathological thought is a kind of inner "air pollution" that alters all the conditions of life in the universe.

In contrast, cleanliness of thought, belief, love, and reciprocity create beneficial frequencies that - fortunately for us - safeguard the universe and fortify it against all the negative forces at work in it.

It is very easy to feel these energies when we are in the presence of a teacher, a spiritual guide, or a "holy man," or in a place that contains spiritual strength and sanctity. Suddenly, all the people who are present in the place are filled with a feeling of love, peace, and reciprocity, without a rational or intellectual understanding of where those feelings came from.

This is the action of an especially powerful magnetic field that encompasses enlightened people or places like those mentioned above. These people transmit positive messages - sometimes without even doing anything - with the help of the electro-magnetic field, their aura, which disseminates and transmits the messages of love and peace, and affects the people in its vicinity.

Methods of strengthening the aura

The stronger, more balanced, and freer of energetic blockages and holes our aura is, the greater our ability to cope with negative external influences, as well as with negative internal ones. A weak electro-magnetic field is liable to cause symptoms of fatigue, listlessness, a greater susceptibility to dominant external energies, frequent mood swings, difficulties with coping, and many other serious problems.

The problem of an electro-magnetic field with a low resonance is noticeable mainly when a person is in the vicinity of dominant and influential people. This is liable to cause him to absorb their influence, opinions, way of life, behavior, and even various personal characteristics. Frequently, when we point out that a certain person has a "strong personality," that person in fact has a strong and forceful aura (but not necessarily a balanced one). The opposite is true when we talk about a person with a "weak personality" (and in most cases, his aura is not balanced). For this reason, it is very important to strengthen the aura and protect it.

There are many different methods for strengthening the aura. Each person must find the methods that suit him and induce a feeling of calmness, pleasantness, and inner strength - a combination of tranquillity and power - in him. It is amazing how simple and natural these "methods" are.

Often, the simplest things that give the person pleasure and cause him to do them intuitively are the ones that strengthen his electro-magnetic field in the most effective manner, increasing and fortifying it.

Being in natural surroundings

Many people feel that being in natural surroundings, passively - sitting near a river, watching the sunset, sitting among trees - or actively - walking, mountain-climbing, swimming in a river, running through a field of flowers - causes them to feel stronger, satisfied, and fulfilled. Gardening and looking at plants also contribute to the strengthening of the aura. Being in natural surroundings and linking up with nature cleanse the aura, fill the person with positive energy, and balance the energies. It is worth trying out several ways of linking up with nature, and finding the one that suits you the most.

Animals

Many people have discovered that their auras can be greatly strengthened by associating with animals they love, taking care of them, petting them, and playing with them. It is nice to look at the aura of a person who is petting his dog lovingly and wholeheartedly, because it is possible to see his aura getting stronger along with a beneficial effect on the animal's aura. There are people who get a deep, almost meditative feeling of calmness from the experience of petting an animal.

Recent studies have shown that keeping an animal in the home is helpful in reducing the incidence of heart disease and in lowering the residents' level of stress and nervousness. One of the ways in which this mechanism works is through a feeling of relaxation on the one hand, and a feeling of connecting and the awakening of affection on the other - two factors that influence the body's systems (mainly through the nervous system) and strengthen the aura. There are people who become filled with energy when they romp wildly and happily with their pets, running and playing with them. (It is amazing to what extent happiness is one of the most beneficial factors regarding the aura!) This behavior even leads to a certain level of energetic balance.

If you are among the people who want to strengthen their auras, you must permit yourself the experience of keeping a pet, and devote beneficial quality time to both of you.

Laughter, happiness, and positive emotions

Laughter and happiness, gaiety and enthusiasm, all strengthen the aura significantly. Happiness is one of the factors that is most beneficial to the aura, and people with the ability to see auras can detect far-reaching changes in the aura of a person when he is happy, or laughs heartily and freely. Happiness begins with a light-hearted and cheerful perception of the world. It is possible to relate to everything with a smile, with acceptance, with resignation, and sometimes even with laughter. Of course, this does not mean that one should laugh in circumstances in which laughter is inappropriate.

Many people discover within themselves - during a heated argument, for example - the ability to look at things from the side, and to free themselves temporarily of personal involvement. Sometimes this puts the incident into such a ridiculous light that they can laugh and discard the burden of negative emotions.

As a rule, positive feelings and emotions such as happiness, love, laughter, compassion, friendship and so on increase the electro-magnetic field substantially, and strengthen and balance it. It is no coincidence that when people are in love, they may suddenly feel full of life and self-confidence, as well as a kind of strength and beneficial power. Happiness, love, laughter, and the rest of the joyful and magnanimous emotions make the aura resonate in a broad range of colors. These emotions cleanse the aura and balance the energetic centers, all the while strengthening the life energy and general health.

It is well known that the more positively and joyfully a person - whose age and state of health are immaterial - relates to life, the healthier and stronger he feels (as opposed to a person whose attitude is not optimistic). When a person is happy, or even only smiles, the change and increase in his electro-magnetic field - even if they are momentary - can be seen.

Singing and dancing

Such simple activities! We're not referring to singing in an opera, or dancing classical ballet. Everyone can burst into song in the shower or while cleaning the house, and dance uninhibitedly to the sounds of the rhythmic or melodious music issuing from the radio. We don't have to waste space writing about the beneficial effect of singing and dancing on the aura and on the entire physical, mental, and spiritual organism.

It should be pointed out that dancing and singing served as mystical, purifying, and energizing tools in many different cultures. Nowadays, these activities are used to strengthen the aura, fill ourselves with energies, divest ourselves of negative loads, and achieve physical, mental, and spiritual balance using many and varied healing techniques, ranging from equilibrium with the help of sounds to dynamic meditation. Every movement and sound has a strong energetic significance and a substantial energetic action. Certain actions induce calmness, while others lead to energetic stimulation, and so on.

It is important to liberate our bodies and voices, but without performing harsh or artificial movements, or using "negative" music such as certain musical styles that aim to give vent to aggression and depression, and originate in polluted places.

Helping others

Relating to other people with love, compassion, understanding, openness, volunteering, and genuine heartfelt help causes the aura to glow and become stronger. Helping others - and again, not in order to be admired, or to coddle our ego, etc. - has a tangible and obvious effect on the karmic aura, and it is one of the wisest ways of solving problems and fixing short-circuits in this aura. Of course, helping others grants us the ability to "get out of ourselves," that is, to free ourselves of the narrow and egocentric perception of the world, to see things in a more correct proportion, and to develop an objective sense. Moreover, it is a springboard to higher spiritual development, and fosters mental and spiritual growth.

It is not a cliche to say he who helps is also helped, and that he who contributes, gains. Those are existential facts. Every truly heartfelt act of volunteering or helping and assisting others has its tangible and immediate reward - first and foremost by the significant strengthening and balancing of the electro-magnetic field that surrounds each one of us.

Furthermore, acts of volunteering and assistance (and this refers to even the "simplest" and "smallest" things) tend to balance the energetic centers (chakras) and the colors of the aura very substantially.

Love

Although this declaration may seem very simplistic, love is the strongest universal energy. Love is capable of strengthening everybody's aura field. Sending love (by means of healing, Reiki, and so on) even to terminally ill or comatose people has been shown to have a powerful effect. True, heartfelt, unconditional love, in every one of its forms (thought, speech, touch) and in every one of its kinds (between the members of a couple, between the members of a family, between friends, the love of a child, of an animal, of the universe, and of every other thing) has an absolutely astonishing effect on the strengthening of the person's electro-magnetic field.

Many healers, experienced and novice alike, as well as people who are not involved with healing in a "conscious" way, have described cases in which the "sending" of love - even from long distances, by the power of thought - inspired good and wonderful feelings in the recipients, even if they were unaware that love had been "sent" to them.

One of the simplest ways of sending love is to sit quietly, empty ourselves of thoughts, fill up with the universal energy of love, which is found in abundance and is accessible to everyone, and imagine that it is passing through us and reaching the person who needs it. Of course, when the universal energy of love passes through us, we also benefit! Every time we think lovingly about a person we love, the energy affects his aura, and strengthens and empowers it - and simultaneously also strengthens our aura.

A friend of mine, a woman of close to eighty, is in the habit of blessing her home every day, and sending love to all the objects and animals in it (as well as to all her friends and acquaintances). Astonishingly, during the twenty years in which she has made a point of doing this, not one electrical appliance in her house has broken down, and she has not had any problems in her house. Moreover, despite her advanced age, and because of her *joie de vivre*, her healthy and balanced way of life, the enormous natural love she has for all the creatures of the universe, and her ability to forgive things wholeheartedly, she is blessed with incredible physical health, a lucid and brilliant mind, and a life filled with vitality and happiness.

Meditation

Meditation is a state in which the brain "takes a rest" from all thoughts and emotions, and focuses on one idea or object. Some meditative states lead the person's brain to alpha waves, a state in which the brain functions at a different speed and at a higher sensitivity of absorption than in its regular waking state. In addition to its significant contribution to the health of the body and mind and to creating a healthy and tranquil life, meditation is known to release tension, dispel negative emotions, increase creativity, and improve the ability to concentrate and focus; it also contributes to spiritual openness to a very great extent.

Meditation can strengthen the aura in a number of ways.

First of all, by getting the person into a state of calmness, meditation exerts a positive effect on the nervous system, muscle tone, blood pressure and circulation, and organ function. When the body becomes stronger and the action of its organs becomes balanced, the aura of the body and the flow in the meridians become stronger, affecting, of course, all the layers of the aura. This is the primary and most basic action of meditation.

In addition, meditation is one of the most excellent tools for development, spiritual growth, filling up with energy, strengthening and cleansing the aura, receiving messages, and developing spiritual abilities such as the ability to sense and see auras.

There is a large variety of methods of meditation that are suitable for different purposes, ranging from calming the body to channeling and receiving messages from divine beings. Basically, most of the forms of meditation include conscious breathing (concentrating on breathing, and different breathing techniques), relaxing the body, or activating it in a particular and conscious way, intellectual calmness, and focusing and centering on what is being done until the mind has been emptied of all emotions and thoughts (in some forms of meditation).

There are methods that concentrate on meditating with certain mantras, and on focusing on the organs of the body or the chakras; there are forms of dynamic meditation in which there is movement; there is meditation to sounds, hypnotic meditation, and numerous other forms of meditation. The vast majority of the various forms of meditation strengthen the body's electro-magnetic field significantly.

Because personality structure varies from person to person, a form of meditation that suits one person is liable to be completely unsuitable for another. This is why each person must carefully check which form of meditation is suitable for him, and not insist too much upon a form that is unsuitable for his personality structure at a given time.

Furthermore, it is important to pay attention to the place in which the meditation takes place. It should be remembered that during meditation, the person's sensitivity to reception is very high. If a person meditates in a place in which there were previously low or negative energies of any kind (and they may still be present there), those energies are liable to penetrate his electro-magnetic field and harm it, especially if he is not experienced and skilled at meditating.

The duration of the meditation is something that must be taken into account, and the person must know the limits of his abilities. When a person who is just beginning to meditate exceeds the boundaries of his meditative abilities, it is similar to a beginner athlete who runs a distance that exhausts his body and his muscles. For this reason, it is important to start meditating for short periods - five to ten minutes - and gradually increase the length of time.

Following is a specific method of meditation that serves to strengthen the aura.

Protective meditation and strengthening the aura

This form of meditation is extremely simple, and even novices can perform it without worry. Despite its simplicity, its effect on the aura is very significant.

Besides strengthening the aura, perseverance in meditating is likely to contribute to the ability to sense and seeing one's own aura, and then gradually other people's auras.

It is not a good idea to eat a heavy meal before meditation. You should drink a little water, and go to the bathroom if necessary.

The meditation should take place in a physically and energetically clean and pleasant room. This is especially important for novices. People who are more experienced in meditation can use their own powers to feel whether the place they are in is suitable for performing meditation or not.

Moreover, it is a good idea to decide upon a fixed place in the home for performing meditation, since the place will gradually absorb the meditative energies that are transmitted in it, and the vibrations there will help the person enter a meditative state more quickly and easily.

Incense, an essential oil burner, or crystals can be placed in the room, but none of these is necessary for this type of meditation. The meditation is performed standing up. Facing the east is considered very beneficial.

The first stage is relaxing the body. Stand with your legs slightly apart, shake your feet, your calves, and your thighs with light movements. Twist your pelvis with loose, circular movements. Shake your hands and arms, and swing your shoulders, your neck, and your head with light, loose movements.

The second stage is emptying your mind of thoughts. Close your eyes, and begin to take deep, calm, and comfortable breaths, ensuring that your breaths are deep enough to fill your entire abdomen (abdominal breathing, not chest breathing). Let your mind empty itself of all thoughts, and concentrate on breathing.

The third stage is filling up with energy. Now you must see a line of white or golden light descending from above, and entering the crown of your head. The white or golden light passes through your spinal column, fills all your organs with light, and then descends via the spinal column to your feet, and penetrates the bowels of the earth.

The fourth stage is strengthening the aura. Now you must see the light ascending from the bowels of the earth, and surrounding your body with a large ellipse of light. You must breathe deeply to the ellipse (this ellipse is the aura) and from the ellipse to you.

This type of meditation is most effective for strengthening the electro-magnetic field, and should be performed before any event that requires any kind of effort, before performing various healing actions, and if there is a feeling of weakness or a lack of energy.

Another method for strengthening the aura

\# Stand with your legs slightly apart; shake your feet, your calves, and your thighs with light movements.

\# Twist your pelvis with loose, circular movements. Shake your hands and arms, and swing your shoulders, your neck, and your head with light, loose movements.

\# When your body feels more relaxed and loose, empty your mind of thoughts, close your eyes and take deep, calm, and comfortable abdominal breaths, all the while concentrating on breathing.

\# Lift your arms straight up, and begin to lower them slowly, being aware that you are strengthening your electro-magnetic field. Your palms must be straight and open, but without any gaps between the fingers.

\# With your palms facing downward, move them slowly downward, until your arms are in line with your shoulders, and continue going down slowly, being aware of the feeling in your palms. (You may be able to feel a kind of "air" or a very delicate substance around you. This is the electro-magnetic field.)

\# While you are moving your hands downward and concentrating on the sensation in them, see the electro-magnetic field that surrounds you becoming stronger in your mind's eye.

\# Continue in this way until your hands are parallel to your thighs, but at a slight distance from them.

\# Repeat the action several times. Remember that the more you perform the action slowly and with greater concentration, the greater the chance that you will be able to feel your electro-magnetic field around you.

This technique should also be performed before any activity that requires effort (physical, mental, or spiritual), before encountering certain people - in whose presence you are inclined to feel uncomfortable - and after the encounter, as well as any time you feel the need for energetic reinforcement.

Cleansing the aura

As we indicated previously, our electro-magnetic field is affected by many different factors, among them external factors. After being in a place that is energetically unclean, after an encounter with people or places with non-positive energy, and every time there is a feeling of a lack of energetic cleanliness, it is important to take steps to cleanse the aura.

These actions are very important for people who spend a lot of time working with appliances that emit radiation (such as computers, microwave ovens, and even TV sets), or being in their vicinity, and especially for practitioners of all kinds.

In every therapeutic interaction, some kind of situation of energetic "identification" is liable to arise, and when you work with people on releasing emotions, anger, and so on - as is the case in psychological treatments and various mental therapies; and on energetic release, as in many healing and alternative medicine techniques - a portion of the negative energies (or more than that, especially if the practitioner's aura is not strong, and he is inclined to identify strongly with his patients) is liable to reach him. For this reason, aura protection and strengthening techniques before the treatment, as well as post-treatment cleansing are absolutely essential, and should not be neglected. (Many practitioners will attest to this!)

Among the simplest and best-known methods for cleansing the aura of non-positive energies, it is important to mention showering and washing hands.

\# A cold shower, which, as we know, also tends to balance the vital state of the body, as well as relax and release it, cleanses the electro-magnetic field well, if not always sufficiently.

Washing hands with the conscious intention of cleansing and purifying the electro-magnetic field, also helps significantly in cleansing the electro-magnetic field.

It is interesting to point out that the aim of washing hands in the morning, according to the Jewish and Islamic traditions, is not for physical cleanliness, but for an energetic cleansing of residual negative energy that is liable to reach the body during the course of the night, when, according to Judaism, the soul levitates during sleep, and the body is left exposed and unprotected energetically.

Following are two additional methods - extremely simple but very effective - for cleansing the aura.

Cleansing the aura using incense

This is an easy and effective method for cleansing the aura, and it is used mainly after treating another person, after a quarrel or a row, after a long, hectic day, and when there is a feeling that non-positive energies have adhered to the aura. The cleansing is performed by a partner, who holds the incense stick. After performing this cleansing frequently with your partner, you may well be able to do so by yourself.

For the cleansing, you can use any stick of natural and quality incense. (There are low-quality incense sticks that are scented with artificial perfumes, and are used for freshening rest-rooms, walk-in closets, and so on - they should not be used.)

The most recommended types of incense are sage (later on we will give instructions for making home-made incense from sage - very strong and effective for purification), frankincense, and jasmine. However, any other stick of good-quality, pleasant-smelling incense is suitable.

Stand up straight, legs slightly apart, and close your eyes. Make sure that you take deep, slow, and comfortable abdominal breaths.

Your partner holds the lit and smoking incense stick, and begins to move it around your body.

There are many different ways of moving the incense stick, but the circular movements should be made from right to left - clockwise.

It is possible to begin from above, and move the incense stick around the head, at a distance of eight to twenty-four inches from the body, in a clockwise direction, gradually descending, in a kind of spiral, to the feet, and then ascending once more.

Another way is to begin on the right side of the body, go down to the feet very slowly, and come up the left side of the body, then go down the right side once more, and up the left side again.

In this technique, intuition and emotions are very important, and if your partner feels that a slightly different way of moving the incense stick is suitable, it is worth trying.

This technique is simple and quick, not to mention very effective. After the cleansing, there is often a feeling of relief and purification (like the feeling of taking a heavy load off one's shoulders), more vitality, and a significant feeling of tranquillity.

Preparing sage incense

In order to prepare sage incense, you need fresh stems (not leaves) of any kind of sage that are covered with many small leaves. The sage plant, with its slightly hairy gray-green leaves, grows in many gardens, and it should be planted in the garden, because its leaves are excellent for many different uses, such as herbal tea for all kinds of complaints, especially stomach-aches. In any case, for preparing incense, you must not use sage that has been picked without permission. It goes without saying that one must not pick any plant from another person's garden without requesting permission; however, when it is a question of preparing incense for cleansing - even if the sage is picked from your own garden - not asking permission impairs its effectiveness from the energetic point of view.

In order to prepare the incense, you need ten to fifteen leafy stems, four to six inches in length. The leaves must be removed from the bottom inch or so of the stem. You should place the leafy stems on the windowsill in the sun so that they dry out a bit, and will subsequently be easier to light. All the stems must be bunched together, and tied up firmly with a piece of white sewing thread. It is very important for the thread to be tight, with no spaces between the stems. After tying them, a thick, fragrant incense stick is formed. After preparing the incense, it should be placed in the sun for a few hours so as to dry out a bit more.

The incense stick should be lit with a lighter or a match, until its end blackens and begins to give off smoke. The smell is pleasant and a bit sharp, and is wonderful for the energetic purification of all the rooms in the house, as well as for cleansing the aura. Sometimes the incense stick goes out after a few minutes, in which case it should be lit again, but in general, the amount of smoke and the fragrance that are produced are sufficient. It is possible to use the same incense stick for a long time.

Cleansing the aura using the "brushing" technique

In this technique of cleansing the aura, you have to use your palm or the back of your hand to "brush" and rub every part of your body vigorously. Start with your head and face, paying special attention to your hair (it must be loosened and fluffed out beforehand), and you must pass your fingers through it and shake it. It is very important to tune in to the fact that you are cleansing your body and aura of all kinds of defective or negative energy. Afterwards, gently move your palms over your face, with the movement from the center of your face outward, as if removing dust. Using light movements, go down to your neck, and from there to your shoulders, with more vigorous movements, as if you were removing dust from your shoulders (exactly as you would do if you were removing lint from your clothes). Continue using vigorous movements down along your arms to your fingertips, directing the negative energy downward, toward the bowels of the earth. Rub your chest and abdomen forcefully, using downward brushing movements, then brush your back (to the best of your ability; places you cannot reach should be cleansed using your thoughts!), your bottom, the inner and outer sides of your thighs and calves, all with vigorous downward movements, until you reach your feet, when you tune in to the thought of sending the negative or defective energies downward, deep into the bowels of the earth.

After you have vigorously "brushed" your whole body, you must shake your hands well and imagine, in your mind's eye, a stream of cool water rinsing them, and "cleansing" them in the purifying jet of water.

Afterwards, with gentle, slow movements, and slow, conscious breaths, move the palm of your hand slowly over your body at a distance of an inch or so from it, trying to feel the field of the aura. Start above your head, slowly go down both sides of your body, including the inner side of your arms and legs, left, right, front and back (where you cannot reach, imagine that you are moving the negative energy downward). You end next to your feet, imagining that you are pushing the negative energy downward, deep into the bowels of the earth.

This cleansing technique brings about an energetic feeling and tranquillity and calmness simultaneously, and it can - and even should - be applied to animals, Of course, you must pay attention to their feelings and reactions.